Why Doctors Are Killing You

by John Hildreth Atkins

Copyright

ISBN
978-1-7947-0984-3

Dedication

This is affectionately dedicated to my lovely bride. She is as pretty today as the day I met her. She deserves better than I can give and I am most thankful that she remains in my life. Hopefully for a long time to come.

Table of Contents

Introduction..page 007
My Nightmare Begins......................................page 017
The Nightmare Continues...............................page 027
Reasons for Blowing up Courthouse.............page 043
Doctors are Killing Covid Patients................page 055
Clues...page 067
"Lack of doctor/patient Relationship"...........page 077
The Tests...page 099
Medical Malpractice & Negligence ....page 113
Education verses Experience..........................page 129
Patient to Doctor..page 139
The Truth About Coronaviruses.................. ..page 167
Why You Must Die...page 187

Introduction

Had my own doctor(s) not been trying to kill me, I might have succumbed to the notion that there really was a pandemic underfoot. I can tell you right here, right now, without any reservation at all, that this whole pandemic is the greatest crime ever perpetrated on mankind (in its' entirety).

Normally, the news would expose such a high-level fraud. But the media is largely controlled by the organized crime family responsible for all of this, and you only hear what they want you to hear (Just look at what Zuckerberg is doing on Facebook to censor us, and Congress supports this censorship)...and I promise you, they do not want you to hear the truth. Are you ready?

Facebook is a social media. What that means is, that people congregate there with other friends and like-minded people. It is NOT a news site. Let me repeat that for you hard-headed sonsofbitches that believe in censorship. It is not a news site and does not require either censorship or regulation. It is an insult to Jews and non-Jews alike to have somebody dictating who we can associate with and what we can talk about.

The nice thing about the internet is that it is like reading a book. If you do not like what is written, you can always turn the page. Only Nasi's and organized criminals censor things. It is tantamount to burning books. Anybody here remember a

7

little piece of crap named Hitler? Question is: if the Jews really hate the Nazis as much as they claim, why do they emulate them so much?

Secondly, proving the pandemic is a fake is as easy as buttering a slice of bread. I will be proving every aspect throughout this book, but I know you are seeking a quick reveal that would leave you to believe me. Okay, let's look at something they are pretty sure you have not paid attention to.

The following is a list of the total deaths in the United States from 1990 through 2020, inclusive. No, these are not covid deaths. These are the total deaths for each successive year.

1990........2.15 million
1991........2.17 million
1992........2.18 million
1993........2.27 million
1994........2.28 million
1995........2.31 million
1996........2.32 million
1997........2.31 million
1998........2.34 million
1999........2.39 million
2000........2.40 million
2001........2.42 million
2002........2.44 million
2003........2.45 million
2004........2.40 million
2005........2.45 million
2006........2.43 million
2007........2.42 million
2008........2.47 million
2009........2.44 million

2010........2.47 million
2011........2.52 million
2012........2.54 million
2013........2.60 million
2014........2.63 million
2015........2.71 million
2016........2.74 million
2017........2.81 million
2018........2.84 million
2019........2.85 million
2020........estimated at 3.1 million

If you are, at all, intelligent, you would have noticed that there was a steady increase in deaths. This increase closely parallels the annual increase in population (births). In other words, looking at these numbers, there is absolutely no sign whatsoever of the alleged pandemic. No evidence.

The next set of numbers comes from the CDC (Center for Disease Control). These are the monthly deaths for the year 2020. Except for a minor "spike" in April, the numbers remained relatively the same all year. What is your yardstick?

You will note the numbers for January and February. This, according to the CDC, was before the pandemic began in the United States. Moreover, the numbers are approximately the same as the numbers reported for 2019. Let's look at the death toll for 2020.

January........264,000 deaths
February......244,000 deaths
March..........269,000 deaths
April............322,000 deaths
May.............280,000 deaths
June.............249,000 deaths

July...............277,000 deaths
August.........274,000 deaths
September...253,000 deaths

At the time I wrote this part of the book, it was March 13, 2021. The numbers were current (as posted on the CDC website). So we do not yet know what the numbers will be for October, November, and December. But rest assured that the CDC is busy trying to "cook the books" in an effort to make it look like a pandemic has been upon us. But even their feeble efforts are futile as there is no evidence of a pandemic and it is nearly impossible to create one out of thin air.

By adding up the data for the months they did give us, we have a total of 2,432,000 deaths. They estimated 3.1 million would have succumbed by 2021. When you subtract the 2,432,000 from 3,100,000, we get 668,000 deaths they figure will have occurred in the missing three months. Divided by three, 222,666 deaths per month for the missing three months. Those are lower than the rest of the year (as shown above). If they intend to try to convince us that there is/was a pandemic, they're going to have to step it up.

An interesting aspect of the CDC is that it only controls information in the United States. Thank God for that. BTW, the head of the CDC is a person named Walensky (see a pattern yet?). So let's take a peek at some things that the CDC can't lie about. Let's look at China and Italy; two hotspots that were in the news for over a year. Is there any evidence of a pandemic there?

The following are the yearly death stats for China. These come from a website called www.macrotrends.net. Let's look for the obligatory spike in deaths that always accompanies a pandemic. Note that these stats list the number of people per thousand that died. I do not have the time nor the desire to look up populations for each year and do the math. Feel free.

1990........6.700 per 1000
1991........6.699 per 1000
1992........6.697 per 1000
1993........6.695 per 1000
1994........6.690 per 1000
1995........6.685 per 1000
1996........6.680 per 1000
1997........6.675 per 1000
1998........6.670 per 1000
1999........6.665 per 1000
2000........6.660 per 1000
2001........6.655 per 1000
2002........6.650 per 1000
2003........6.645 per 1000
2004........6.686 per 1000
2005........6.727 per 1000
2006........6.767 per 1000
2007........6.808 per 1000
2008........6.849 per 1000
2009........6.880 per 1000
2010........6.911 per 1000
2011........6.941 per 1000
2012........6.972 per 1000
2013........7.003 per 1000
2014........7.027 per 1000
2015........7.050 per 1000
2016........7.074 per 1000
2017........7.097 per 1000
2018........7.121 per 1000
2019........7.261 per 1000
2020........7.402 per 1000

2021........7.542 per 1000

As you can plainly see, there was no noticeable spike in deaths in China. This defies logic and the United States will cry foul. So let's take a look at the other hotspot; Italy. Again, this is the number of people per thousand.

1990........9.649 per 1000
1991........9.680 per 1000
1992........9.712 per 1000
1993........9.744 per 1000
1994........9.777 per 1000
1995........9.811 per 1000
1996........9.844 per 1000
1997........9.878 per 1000
1998........9.911 per 1000
1999........9.887 per 1000
2000........9.863 per 1000
2001........9.839 per 1000
2002........9.815 per 1000
2003........9.791 per 1000
2004........9.781 per 1000
2005........9.770 per 1000
2006........9.760 per 1000
2007........9.749 per 1000
2008........9.739 per 1000
2009........9.815 per 1000
2010........9.892 per 1000
2011........9.968 per 1000
2012.......10.045 per 1000
2013.......10.121 per 1000
2014........10.192per 1000
2015.......10.262 per 1000

2016.......10.333 per 1000
2017.......10.403 per 1000
2018.......10.474 per 1000
2019.......10.566 per 1000
2020.......10.658 per 1000
2021.......10.749 per 1000

Isn't it interesting how every country in the world can tell you an accurate death rate, but not the United States? They even have the death rate for this year (so far this year). But the United States cannot even tell us how many people died in October, November, and December of 2020? Something is very wrong.

I think that it is more than obvious that the United States is waiting to "pad" the numbers to try to convince us that we are in the midst of some pandemic. As we move through this book, I will be proving every aspect of this scheme. I will give you motive, method, a simple cure, a preventative, and the truth. All will shock you as it is organized crime at its worst.

To better understand this, we first need to take a quick look at what, exactly, constitutes a pandemic. According to the Oxford dictionary, a pandemic is "a disease that is prevalent over a whole country or the world." Obviously, this is not an acceptable definition because, under that premise, the common cold is a pandemic. We definitely need something a little more substantial. After all, the bastards did lock us up and took away our Rights.

Webster's defines pandemic as "an outbreak of a disease that occurs over a wide geographic area (such as multiple countries or continents) and typically affects a significant proportion of the population." Therein lies the rub. At what point does an epidemic become a legitimate pandemic? Clue:

"affects a significant proportion of the population."

As a child, we all learned about the Trojan Horse. That was a story about how some sneaky bastards built a giant wooden horse so their cohorts could hide inside of it. They then gave the horse to their enemies as a peace offering. Their enemies took the horse inside their fort where, under the cover of darkness, the sneaks crept out and slaughtered their enemies.

More recently, we have all heard about the 1938 radio broadcast wherein a not-so-jovial Orson Welles scared the hell out of listeners by announcing that alien spacecraft had landed and were slaughtering humans at will. Though it was even announced as a radio teleplay, people panicked; many even went so far as to kill themselves.

Fear is a horrible thing. It does not take much for someone to scare another person. For instance, all one has to do is to wait until we're in the middle of another cold/flu season and announce that the dirty Chinese had manufactured a new virus and that virus had escaped from a laboratory in Wuhan. That is all it took.

We have all seen movies and been bombarded with newspapers and television publishing reports that outlined the risks and horrors of experimenting with microscopic organisms. Remember the uproar over Dolly? Dolly was a sheep that was cloned from another. OMG, they're playing Gods now!

To reinforce the lie about the escaped virus, we were shown films of the Chinese locking people in their homes and spraying down the streets. Each of us drew the same conclusion: if it didn't happen just as Uncle Sam was saying, why were the Chinese going through such extremes to fight it off?

Yes, I know, you are set in your ways. The twelve years

that they brainwashed you (in school) have convinced you that you should be loyal to the United States government. You mistakenly believe that we and the government are one and the same. Hell no. Not just no, but hell no! We aren't.

The American government is run by thugs with an agenda that has nothing at all to do with either you or me. It is as cruel and evil as any on the face of the Earth. By the time you finish this book, you will know that I speak the truth.

One question that should be in your mind is, if they went so far as to market a fake pandemic, what else did they do? I cannot hardly wait to tell you but let's take a look at what they did to me first. In this way, we can get a chronological order of just how medical malpractice morphed into an all-out pandemic. You're not going to believe it, but it's all true and just as I say it is. What's more, the things they have done to me, they are doing to elderly and infirmed people all over the planet. If you are at all squeamish, my advice for you is to put this book down. Some things you just shouldn't know.

My Nightmare Begins

I considered leaving out this part of my story because of the negative connotations associated with it. Unfortunately, such an omission is not an option as my enemies will bring it up in a fervent effort to discredit everything I say. Please keep that in mind as I expose the whole sordid story. More importantly, look at the facts, even as you know them, and ask yourself what the truth is.

I have written and published more than fifty books. One book got an innocent man out of prison after the poor sap spent 30 years there for a murder that he, not only did not commit but, was framed for...by his own lawyer(s), the D.A., the Cops, the Attorney General, and Judges. That book is called "Prosecuting the Prosecution." In case you want to read just how corrupt your local government is.

After I successfully helped free Frank Gable from prison, people asked me what true crime I was going to write about next? I had no idea...until someone suggested that I tackle the assassination of President John F. Kennedy.

I must admit, I balked at the idea of looking into the JFK thing...simply because so many years had passed that I was sure that somebody must have figured it out. Like so many others, I was content just to accept that Lee Harvey Oswald did it; or, at the very least, had some part in it. But then I looked at the Zapruder film. Oh-oh.

It took me a mere thirty seconds to figure out who really killed JFK. I suggest you go to youtube and look for yourself. But knowing who killed Kennedy did not solve all of the riddles. I would spend better than a year reading testimony, looking at documents, searching through photographs, as well as numerous visits to mapquest.

How was it that I could solve the riddle of who killed Kennedy so quickly? Actually, it was as simple as drawing a hot knife through butter. I merely asked the obvious question: If Zapruder was there to film the President, why wasn't the President in the video?

As you go through this book, keep asking the obvious questions. The first should be, why am I writing this expose? Why am I opposing organized crime? Your second question should be, am I crazy? And now we come to that part of the story.

In 1974, I was framed for a burglary of a hardware store. Though I had no criminal record outside of a juvenile record for drinking alcohol and violating curfew, in 1975, I was sentenced to 10 years in prison. Sounds harsh and you would be right. So the question begs, why was I wrongly convicted and such a lengthy sentence imposed when virtually all first offenders were getting probation?

The short answer is because the authorities were afraid of me. I was rumored to have stolen ten cases of 70 grade dynamite. More rumors abounded wherein I was allegedly plotting to blow up the Polk County Courthouse in Dallas, Oregon. And why would anyone want to do such a dastardly deed? Government corruption. Crooked bastards.

So now the stage is set. I was twenty-one when they sent me to prison. Ten years was a long time to sit without making money and so I engaged in numerous venues for accruing some measure of financial gain. That was how it came to be that the older cons revealed to me that I could go on disability and draw a monthly check of some three hundred dollars.

Let me tell you, that pittance might seem trite to you, but in 1975, in prison, that was a lot of money. I had no idea how long I would actually be in prison, but I knew that if it was for three or four years, I could save up enough money to buy a house. Yes, there were houses around for under ten thousand in those days.

Problem was, I was not physically handicapped, beyond the fact that I was incarcerated. My new associates reminded me that there was always mental. "But I'm not crazy," I lamented.

"Don't think so?" one of the cons countered. "What do you call it when you have a chance to get rich and you don't take it?"

The old boy was absolutely correct. It was stupid to just sit inside and do nothing. After all, the Polk County authorities did their best to convince a judge and jurors that I was totally mad. Why not use that to my benefit? Why leave prison a broke bastard?

I tried various schemes to get sent to the nut ward. One was shaving my head and painting crosses on my face. That plan backfired when some of the younger cons did likewise. I'm not sure why they did that but I am guessing that it had something to do with rebelling against the system. They knew it worried the guards.

I had just about given up on the notion when an event placed me in the perfect position to "go upstairs." PSU, the Prison Psychiatric Unit, was upstairs. I was downstairs, in S & I (Segregation and Isolation, referred to as "the building"). I had managed to get put into the building by shoving the block sergeant's desk, and the block sergeant, into the wall of my cell block. Huh?

19

It was summertime, 1976, and I was residing on the fifth tier (floor) of cell block D. It was hot and stinky up there. But that wasn't precisely the reason why I had requested to go up there in the first place. You see, the woman's prison was just over the wall that separated us. I knew that, if I went up to the top tier, I would be able to see the girls. I would also be able to see the girls that walked by on the street below. Unfortunately, I was placed at the wrong end of the tier and I couldn't see a damned thing.

To say I hated it would be an understatement. Though I was in great shape, I still had to walk up and down five flights of stairs everytime I went to my "house;" (my cell). Because I was taking college courses, I had to walk up three more flights of stairs to go to school. It was getting old.

I had gone to the block sergeant to get reassigned to a cell down on the third tier. He had reassured me that he would move me down when a cell became available. So it was, that on a day when damned near the whole tier was released on parole or whatever, I confronted the man. When he refused to honor his pledge, I pinned his dumbass against the wall with his desk and screamed all manner of obscenities at him.

After the lying bastard blew his rape whistle, the goon squad thundered in and ushered me off to the building. As soon as we got there, they had me stand against a wall while they decided what to do with me. Because, technically, I had assaulted one of them, I was sure there was going to be an ass-whipping involved so I just slumped to the floor and tried to block it out.

The violence I expected never materialized. Instead, they were afraid of me because I wouldn't talk to them. In the interim, they had telephoned Dr. Weissert, the head of the PSU ward. He ordered them to dress me out. That meant changing from my prison blues into an orange jump suit. I was on my way.

I swear, I had no conscious intention of appearing loony. I merely wanted to block the pain I knew was coming. Next thing I knew, I was led up some stairs and into Weissert's office.

Weissert asked me two questions. "Do you ever talk to God?"

Absolutely. I had guardian angels, God, or some kind of divine intervention, that was keeping me safe. I silently spoke to God fairly frequently. But I did not tell him that. Instead, I simply orated, "yes."

His second question was: "Does he ever answer you?"

"Oh, hell yes," I responded enthusiastically, "all the time."

That's it. That was the full extent of our conversation. Two questions. Both of them, innocent enough. Both answered honestly. And that, apparently, was enough to justify what he said next.

"Okay," the good doctor intimated, "I'll certify you, but you have to promise to take your meds the whole time you're in here."

There were meds? Oh, hallelujah. Money _and_ drugs. In that moment, I was the happiest man alive. Save money and get high. In my mind, I was thinking about the fun drugs; things that made a man's time go by so fast that it seemed like days instead of years. But I couldn't have been more mistaken.

Right from the get-go, I abhored those drugs with all my being. Though the years have clouded my recollection of exact dosages, I know that I was placed on Stellazine and, eventually, Melloril. One of those had been bumped up to 400mg and the other had been 800mg. Both sucked.

I was placed in an observation cell with a solid steel door and a small window I could look out of, and vice versa. The cell was located right across from Weissert's office. It featured an elevated concrete slab right in the center. That was my "bed."

I hated those drugs and did pushups and everything else I could think of to do that might expel them from my system. Nothing worked. I was having second thoughts. No amount of money was worth what I was experiencing. But it was too late to back out.

Eventually, they opened my door, probably because I wasn't screaming or banging on anything. This allowed me to mingle with the other patients. What an experience that was.

One guy, I think his name was Roger, used to stand there and occasionally do the "prolixin shuffle." In a way, I actually envied him. His drugs had all but incapacitated him.

An old goat, named Merle, with a long white beard was a bit of an artist. He gave me some materials and let me paint a few pictures. He had a mischievious streak but was a pleasant enough fella.

And then there was Jonesy. This old coot was skinnier than a bean pole and was about as cantankerous as any old person I ever met. He was always grumbling about something and cocking his head to one side to give you the look. As it turned out, that had been Jonesy's last residence. Everybody, staff and inmates, missed him. Whatever else he had been, he was entertaining.

Then came James Ross. I wasn't much older than him but I thought of him as a kid. Maybe he was a little older. I do not remember. He was big, but a kid nonetheless. He came up to me and stated that I did not seem crazy; what was I doing up there?

"I'm here to get a check," I said without thinking.

I regretted saying it the minute it rolled off of my lips. It's one of those "need to know," kind of things. By that time, I already knew that Ross was in for statutory rape. What that meant was that he had been screwing some girl under eighteen. The guy was from Falls City. That wide spot in the road did not have a lot going for it. Basically, if you lived in Falls City, you were drinking beer and trying to screw everything in sight. I had no doubt whatsoever that the sex had been consensual. But Ross was like me, a rebel, and he had pissed off the powers that be.

"What do you mean?" he demanded to know.

It was too late. I had already opened my big mouth. So I explained that Weissert certified people so they could get checks. I quickly added that the doctor would not certify Ross.

"Why not?"

Ross had informed me that he was getting released in a few weeks. So I tried to explain to him that Dr. Weissert would never certify him because there was nothing in it for Weissert. I might as well have been speaking to the wall. Jim already had dollar signs in his head and nothing was going to deter him from his quest. Or so he thought.

Ross made a beeline into Weissert's office. I grimaced with the realization that Ross intended to force Weissert's hand and that could not be good for either of us. I all but ran to my cell and closed the door. As I did, Ross demanded that Weissert get him a check. Weissert looked up and I got the look; a look that was much more menacing than little ol' Jonesy's.

I cringed and crouched down behind the door. Ross was getting louder and more boisterous. Then he made the biggest blunder of his soon-to-be short life. He threatened to tell on Weissert. Oh shit.

Looking back on that moment, I honestly believe that Ross was certifiable. Who in their right mind makes threats against

23

their captors?

Weissert wasted scant time in picking up the telephone and calling the goon squad. And they didn't dilly-dally getting there. Watching from the narrow slot at the bottom of my door, I saw them take Ross down to his final resting place: Segregation and Isolation.

On August 1, 1976, James Ross was found hanging from a sheet in his cell. A hospital orderly revealed that Ross's hands were tied behind his back when they brought him up. His cellmate slept through the whole thing. It was ruled a suicide by the Oregon State police and the Medical Examiner.

Meanwhile, Salem, Oregon, police (where the prison is located) took my little brother to the ground and stuck guns to his head. To this day, he has no idea why. But the message was loud and clear to me.

Weissert never said anything to me; he didn't have to. And I did not bring it up the whole time I was in prison. I would spend 2 years and 2 months inside before getting paroled. And no, I never got my check. After what happened to Ross, I decided I didn't need it. I abruptly stopped taking the drugs when I was released to general population a couple of months later. I endured hell as I withdrew from those drugs, but I was determined not to take them. Think about it.

You see, if I stayed on the drugs, Weissert would have used his clout to keep me inside prison as long as he could. Why? Glad you asked. Each prison has a certain percentage of inmates who are certifiable. My personal opinion is that half of the inmates were certifiable. However, the federal government doesn't see it that way. If Weissert certified a higher percentage of inmates as crazy, the feds might step in and take a look at his operation. So?

You really don't get it, do you? Dr. Weissert was the head of the psyche ward. He was also the head of the Oregon State

Hospital. That's what they call the nut house. It's close to, but separate from, the penitentiary. See? Of course you don't.

Dr. Weissert was able to write checks for virtually anything and for any amount. Aside from controlling inmates at both institutions, he was supposed to oversee the entire operation of each. So even if he did not personally write a check, he could cause one to be written and/or approved.

For every inmate certified in custody, money came in from the feds and/or state of Oregon. This was because, at least in theory, the institutions incurred addition expense caring for crazy people. Weissert considered it free money. Moreover, it was routine business to skim money off of inmates' accounts. That's why Weissert certified inmates and excluded short-timers like James Ross.

My diagnosis? Weissert claimed that I was paranoid schizophrenic because God spoke to me. He equated that to voices in the head. While it's true, there was an occasional voice, when I told him that God answered me all the time, I did not mean voices. God answers in many ways and only an ignorant sonofabitch would ever deny it.

On the other hand, what is wrong with voices? We all hear them. Are you seriously trying to tell me that you do not? You're just not paying attention. Tell me, what does a thought look like? As you are reading this book, there is a tiny little voice, your own, speaking it in your head. Such is the nature of thought. Get over it.

Doctors have not figured it out yet. We all talk to ourselves whenever we read. Now imagine what happens as you grow older and that restraint comes down. Instead of silently talking to yourself, you begin to talk out-loud and people look at you funny. Schizophrenia is not so much that a person is crazy as it is the barrier that silences us breaks down and they speak their minds. Think about it.

25

While you are at it, consider what would have happened if I had stayed on the psyche meds. Eventually, little by little, they would have fried my brain. That is to say, while they might help truly crazy people (by scrambling their brains), the drugs could, and would, eventually destroy parts of my brain. Imagine my chagrin if I appeared before the parole board and I was unable to properly communicate with them. There is a reluctance to let "crazies" out of confinement.

And so it is that I have had to walk a fine line ever since that day. Somewhere, somehow, Weissert had entered his assessment into the record. In later life, after suffering physically in a car accident, I attempted to get disability. The woman who was in charge of making that determination flat told me that she could not certify me physically, but she could mentally. It has been problematic. Thanks, but no thanks.

One more thing, before we continue, there is no cure for schizophrenia. The fact that I do not have it now, nor at any time other than prison, proves that Weissert was up to no good.

The nightmare had begun...but the war was far from over.

The Nightmare Continues

Thankfully, I was released from prison in the summer of 1977. I had gained a lot of experience and learned the kinds of things you cannot derive from a textbook. Each lesson became another layer in the complex world in which I lived. And each layer reinforced my amazement at how corrupt the authorities really were.

The good news, if there truly was any, was that I would no longer need to contemplate blowing things up. I had spent considerable time studying chemistry and ruminating on how best to take on an enemy that had you outgunned, out manned, and owned both the courts and the police. It was disheartening, to be sure. But not insurmountable.

The bad news was that I was branded by a twisted doctor who had no business being in charge of an outhouse, let alone two institutions. To top it all off, as I would eventually discover, the drugs were experimental and had left me sterile. I have no known children...not for want of trying.

Somewhere along the way, I adopted the word recalcitrant. I have no idea where it came from; I only know that it just popped into my head one day and I looked it up. It means stubbornly opposed to authority. You're damned right I am. All authorities are idiots. Recalcitrant.

Now would be a good time to digress for just a minute. By now, I am sure that you believe I stole the dynamite and was hell-bent on blowing up the courthouse. All that you lack is motive. Before you can accuse me, you have to have motive. Let's see if I can provide you with the requisite amount.

In fourth or fifth grade, I decided to try to bond with the other kids by going out for football. I did not know a thing about the game, beyond my father watching it, and had said as much to my teacher/guide. She assured me that it would be okay; the coach would teach me how to play. And so it was, I trotted confidently onto the field.

Imagine my surprise when the quarterback tossed me the ball. I caught it and took off running. But I was not sure I was even going in the right direction. Somehow the other kids figured that out and the opposing team chanted "you're running the wrong way." I abruptly reversed direction, much to the consternation of my teammates.

We had been playing flag football (as opposed to the more familiar tackle football). To end a runner's play, you simply had to tear off a flag that was hanging from his belt. One of my teammates tore mine off; ending the play.

As luck would have it, one of my teammates was mad as hell and punched me in the nose. To make matters worse, the coach balled me out and threw me off of the team. Their opinion had been that I was somehow clowning around. So the question begs, if the opposing team knew I didn't know how to play, why didn't the coach? After all, he had witnessed their telling me I was going the wrong way.

My teacher, a very dear lady, God bless her soul, had been wrong. The coach had been wrong. Virtually every authoritative person in my life had been wrong, from the principal with a spanking fetish to another teacher who once tossed my lunch into the trash so I had to starve that day. Although I had grown accustomed to starving, thanks to an alcoholic father, I was deeply hurt and even more deeply angered at the woman's cold, callous, and unconscionable acts. How dare her.

Let's fast forward, for brevity, to Polk County. My life in Coos Bay, Oregon, had been a nightmare. I had looked forward to life in Dallas, Oregon. But the nightmare was not about to end. Whatever Coos Bay had been, Dallas was worse. Boy was it.

I had been a shy kid; too shy to seriously bond with the other kids. They were an unknown quantity to me. I was a numbers guy. If A equals B, and B equals C, then A must equal C. It's an equation where it does not matter what the value is for any of the letters. Pretty easy to grasp, eh?

According to the Constitution, A (substitute boys) equals B (sub girls) because all are considered equal in the eyes of the law. A equals B. But what about C? What about it?

There is an inclination to assume that C equals mankind. However, that doesn't work because boys do not make up all of mankind; nor do girls make up mankind. In the example, we must add A + B = mankind. If you kick this around using its most fundamental values, it can get pretty confusing; especially if you are one of those who want to factor in race, religion, or any other distraction from the basic precepts.

You know, all of that looks good on paper. Unfortunately, real life does not conform to basic mathematical formulas. Do not discriminate based on age. How ludicrous to suppose that a two year-old should have the same Rights as a 21 year-old. Not sure I want the little sucker drinking up my beer.

Laws are a necessary evil but can, themselves, be evil. It is for this very reason that the law is divided into two parts. In the first part, called the "letter of the law" by those astute people with law degrees, we are all created equal. However, we cannot allow a mother or father to give their babies alcohol to sedate them, so there is another side of the law called the "intent of the law."

Intent of the law. Specifically, the legislative intent of the law. What were the framers of the law trying to aid or prevent when they passed the law? Knowing that there are too many idiots running loose in society, the legislators realized that they could not simply state that we are all equal in the eyes of the law. A thing called common sense mandates that we do not give our children alcohol. And so that was addressed by legislative comment (intent).

All of that still looks pretty good on paper, doesn't it? You are so disillusioned. The fact is, laws do not mean a thing if they are not enforced or they are enforced unfairly. Remember the coach who reprimanded me for no reason instead of addressing the boys who had told me to run the wrong way? And don't forget the kid who assaulted me? On what planet was any of that construed as acceptable behavior; let alone sportsmanlike conduct?

Boys will be boys. Yes sir. That's why they had a coach there. He was supposed to teach everybody how to play the game. He was supposed to teach good conduct and sportsmanship. Above all else, he should have been insuring that kids did not injure other kids.

Now carry all of that into everyday life. Under the legal system, the police enforce the law by making arrests and handing out tickets. Everybody knows that, right? Wrong. While the letter of the law is crystal clear, it is often disregarded. For instance, the letter of the law called for the arrest and incarceration of the kid who punched me in the nose. Following his arrest, he would have been prosecuted by the District Attorney or the D.A.'s assistant. Judgment and sentencing would have been handed down by a Judge and/or Jury.

The system is in place, but it is worthless because some

people are prosecuted and others not. To make matters worse, there is no guarantee that people, especially cops, are not going to lie. Many people really are innocent and yet they sit behind bars. Why? Because the system is more concerned with convicting someone, anyone, than it is in convicting the right people. To make it worse, if you get a group in charge, they can easily say you did something, have a judge sign a paper saying you confessed, or whatever, and sentence you to prison or worse. It happens with unimpeded regularity.

My girlfriend and I had walked downtown to attend a movie. Afterwards, we were walking back to her/our apartment when the police confronted us. Curfew was midnight. As I recall, it was about fifteen minutes after twelve. I was arrested.

First of all, the police had no probable cause to harass us. We were not doing anything but walking home. Secondly, arresting somebody for curfew at 12:15am on a Friday night is almost entirely unheard of. Next thing I know, I'm in Juvenile Detention; locked in a cell the size of a small closet.

I would spend the next two weeks locked up inside that closet before being released back to Polk County from Marion County. The delay had been the result of my father being home. You see, he was a child molester who wanted to molest my sister(s); his own daughter(s). Kind of hard to do when their older brother is around.

I do not remember how long I was in jail in Polk County before they placed me in a foster home in Monmouth (some eight miles from Dallas). My foster parents were an elderly couple who had, more or less, adopted my ten year-old foster brother when he was a baby. Shortly after arriving there, I got a job.

I was fifteen, I was working as a box boy for a major supermarket. I loved my job, in large part because it was the only store in a small college town and most of the students were girls. Besides, my boss was a great guy and the job was super easy...not that I minded hard work. I had actually gotten the job because I had been hired to help unload a truckload of watermelons and I had busted my ass getting it done.

At that point, for the first time in my entire life, everything was good. I had my own car. I was on summer vacation, but was planning on going to school when it started back up. Then my foster brother started demanding that I take him to Dairy Queen.

I am the kind of guy that likes to share the wealth, so-to-speak, and I would take my foster brother up there for ice cream or whatever. But then he became more and more demanding that I do so. Eventually, he tried to blackmail me by saying he was going to go tell our foster parents that I threatened to kill them or some such horseshit.

The little bastard was true to his word and I found myself face to face with my juvenile counselor. My mother had let my father come back after having kicked him out for the umpteenth time or, more than likely, the douchbag merely abandoned her and moved in with his mama again. However it happened, he was back again and fighting to keep me from going there. Only my mother wasn't having any more of his bullshit and the juvvies paroled me home.

Up until a few months before my sixteenth birthday, my entire criminal record had been primarily confined to something like three arrests for minor in possession of alcohol (by consumption) and four arrests for curfew (being out late). Both of these things are things that the police can arrest you for. Usually they don't. This is especially true if they know you're heading home.

I continued to work at the store and bought another car because my old one had caught fire. Between work and hanging out with my friends (all of whom were at least 21), I was not home much; which I'm sure appeased the old man on some level.

In case you're wondering, all of my friends were older because kids my own age seemed so infantile and immature. And so it had been that I did all the things that older people do. We drank beer and often drove around all night. Pretty exciting, huh?

One day, one of my friends needed some empty boxes. So we drove over to the store where I worked and went around back. That's where we threw away all of our discarded boxes and stuff. We rounded up the requisite number of boxes, as well as a case of canned nuts and some magazines. I better explain.

One of the things that stores do is to make sure that everything is fresh and current. Pretty much anything in a package, can, bottle, or otherwise, has an expiration date stamped on it. Whenever we discovered a product that had expired, we tossed it out. So it really wasn't a big deal to find a case of nuts tossed out. Likewise, we frequently tossed out old magazines as the distributors considered it a favor so they didn't have to deal with them.

So we returned to Dallas with our boxes and the stuff we found. I placed the nuts and magazines in the trunk of my old car before going and helping my friend pack.

Several days went by relatively uneventful. Then my father saw me open my trunk and hand my sister a can of nuts. It was the moment he had hoped for...another excuse to get me out of his way. So he called the cops and told them I had stolen the stuff from the store where I worked.

Let's examine the modus operandi, or method of action, for the typical pedophile or predator. Sex offenders will usually use gimmicks and/or bribes to elicit the desired response from their victims. My father was no different. He would offer the girls money, candy, clothes, and even a week at girl scout camp. When he saw me giving them something, it represented one less gimmick for him to use in his sinister quest.

Another trait inherent in predators is that they like to gather information. This means that they snoop, spy on, or otherwise solicit information that will help them in their quest. This adequately explains why my father was in a position to see me get in the trunk of my car (behind the house). Either he had been watching my sister (most likely) or he had been watching me. I never asked and neither did the juvenile authorities. We'll never know.

Week after week, I sat idly in a jail cell. There was no facility in Polk County for juveniles. I cried. I had done nothing wrong. I wanted out to go to work. My boss would have let me. But then how was I to get there? I had a car but no driver's license. My Learner's permit was only legitimate if there was someone eighteen or older in the car. What a dilemma.

Everything could have been straightened out if only someone had listened to me. First of all, I hated nuts; still do. I cannot even tell you if they were peanuts or mixed nuts. Didn't matter to me as I had no intention of eating them. BTW, I still hate nuts, although I kinda like Pistachios, corn nuts, and cashews. But rarely.

My boss could have figured it out if I could have talked to him. He knew I would take stuff I didn't like because he had offered me some watermelons when I unloaded the truck and I told him I didn't like watermelon but took one for my foster parents. That probably sounds conflicting to you but it really isn't. If given to me, I would accept things I did not like. But not steal them.

What about the magazines? I was almost sixteen. What kinds of magazines do you think a teenaged boy liked? Playboys? Yes. Penthouse? Yes. But there weren't any of those. What I had was something like Cosmopolitan and Woman's World. To date, I have not read either of those titles, nor do I ever plan on reading either.

So I'm trying to explain to the police and the juvenile authorities that if I was going to steal anything, it would be something I liked. That was not rocket science. Nor were they rocket scientists. Dumb as stumps.

And so it was I started rebelling in jail. Raising hell and going to the hole. I was not going down without a fight. And what started that? I had been reading law books and discovered that there was a law regarding emancipation. The letter of the law stated that a ten year old boy could be emancipated to help out his family. I was 15...almost 16.

If you are thinking that they refused to emancipate me because of legislative intent, you couldn't be more wrong. The emancipation law was enacted during the Civil War because fathers and older boys went off to fight. Many died and that left the family farm to be run by the widow. By emancipating her younger children (usually boys), this allowed the younger children to stay at home and work instead of going to school.

When they refused to let me call my boss, and they refused to emancipate me, I went ballistic. I was so tired of adults screwing up my life for little or no reason. It just wasn't right. I was losing everything I had worked so hard for.

And so it was that the juvenile authorities decided to give me psyche tests. Part of that process was to try to determine the maturity level of my brain. That is to say, they desired to know how smart I was (or wasn't). You tell me. How many kids (or adults, for that matter) do you know that would read law books in jail instead of laying around watching television?

A big part of the Constitution was to make sure that all people got a fair shake irregardless of their age or sex. Yet I was being discriminated against on the flimsiest of excuses.

After a week of testing, they determined my I.Q. to be in excess of 187. Mentally and maturity-wise, I was more than qualified to be emancipated. Age-wise, I was more than qualified to be emancipated. At no time in history was a young man more qualified to be emancipated. Noone. And yet, it was not to be.

My captors could not prosecute me for a crime they could not prove and so, on September 3, 1969, a Judge sentenced me to reform school for "being out of parental control." No such charge existed either before or after. My Constitutional Right to confront my accusers: this being both my father and, theoretically, my boss, was denied. I had no legal representation.

You probably think that, in their eyes, justice had been served. Not even close. They all knew better. Years later, I found out that my father had gone all-out in molesting my sister(s). I also found out that the reason I was sent to reform school had nothing, whatsoever, to do with anything I may have done. The reason I was put through hell? Foster homes only wanted little girls; none of them wanted teenaged boys. I was being discriminated against because of my gender, as well as my age.

I want you to think about the base principle here. Anytime that a person goes to jail for any significant amount of time, they lose everything they had worked so hard to get. You lose your home, you lose your car, in many cases, you lose your friends, and a myriad of things both tangible and intangible. You are separated from loved ones, family, and the simple ability to enjoy time with them.

If everything had been confined to those loses, my time in reform school might have been tolerable. But it was not meant to be. The other kids, not to mention the staff, were all of the opinion that I was lying about why I was there. After all, there was no such charge as the one I was sentenced with. After being physically and mentally abused, I quickly decided that I needed to make up some excuse for being there. But what?

I was not a bad person. I had not robbed or assaulted anyone. I had stolen nothing. What excuse could I use that would put me in a more favorable light with my peers; if not the authorities? I settled on drugs. I let it be known that I was busted for drugs. It was a risky undertaking as I had no experience at all with drugs...other than I may have smoked pot once.

Some kid even challenged me on the pot thing. I had taken a hit off of a joint. I had no idea what color the pot inside was. After thinking on it a minute, I told the kid it was brown because plants are green before being dried out and turning brown (like tobacco). When the kid chided me by saying I was wrong, that pot was green, a more knowledgeable kid put him in his place.

"That dirt weed you smoke might be green," my defender orated, "but the really good stuff is brown."

I had silently breathed a sigh of relief. I had dodged a bullet. But only one. I had more obstacles in front of me; not the least amongst these was the shrinks I was forced to see.

I can honestly say that there are very few people that I ever wanted to hit as much as I wanted to hit my shrink(s). Try as I may, I could not get them to listen to me. It was so bad that they sat me down and started preaching to me about goals.

"There are long term goals and there are short term goals,"

four-eyes mono-droned.

"Such as?" I demanded.

"Well, you can't stay in your parent's roost forever. You need to start planning on finishing school and going to work and taking care of yourself."

I cannot tell you how much that infuriated me. I jumped to my feet, yelling, "f#$k you. What the hell do you think I was doing when they sent me here?"

They had all been trying to convince me that I was in some sort of denial. I had challenged them to look up my record before they spoke to me again. They refused. Because I was in reform school, I had to be some stupid, lazy, no good bum who thought himself above the law. No sir, that would come later.

When I steadfastly refused to talk to another shrink, they locked me in segregation. The way those idiots saw it, the isolation would compel me to speak with them. Wrong answer. I felt safe in the hole. I did not have to worry about getting beat up or whatever.

In the hole, I read a book a day. I would have read more, but they only let you have one book. That was stupid. I thought the whole point of the "school" was to educate. What better way to learn how to read than to actually do it?

One thing that I liked about the hole was that you were not allowed to talk. I enjoyed the peace and quiet. However, I had a question and yelled out to the guys for an answer. Me and a couple of guys started talking about it. One of the other kids told us to shut up because we weren't supposed to talk.

"Oh really?" I screamed. "What are they going to do; lock us up?"

That got the guys laughing and pretty soon everybody was talking up a storm. I had opened a pandora's box. So much for silent serene solitude.

At some point, one of our captors got the brightest idea ever advanced by a person in a position of authority; this moron took away our books. Of course I felt obligated to educate the dumbass. First I pointed out the fact that kids needed to learn to read. Books were also educational in other ways. And then the obvious began. Without a book to distract them, even the quiet kids started yelling and cussing.

Not sure if the man had wised up or, more than likely, his superiors chastised him for being an idiot. Not only did we get our books back, they even allowed us to have two a day. Variety is nice. I usually grabbed a couple of Reader's Digests. That way I could read the things I liked and, if I got bored, I would read some things that I did not particularly care about. Educational. Win-win.

They eventually let me out of the hole. I never found out why. Maybe they hated me for starting a rebellion in their nice quiet facility. Maybe they realized that I was never going to give in and see the shrinks. Maybe they hired a new guy with some measure of intelligence. Doubtful. The best, most likely, reason is probably because they had a time limit on how long they could detain a juvenile in solitary confinement. Supreme Courts are funny that way.

As I stated earlier, the place was not prepared for someone of my intelligence. Their classrooms only taught stuff that I had, essentially, learned in grade school. Apparently juvvies were retarded or something. That left me two choices. One, I could go to work. I quickly shot that down when I discovered they paid you an extraordinary nothing. Zero. Zilch. Not one red cent. The hole was calling my name.

And so it was that I opted to fill my day with vocational training classes. I learned upholstery, electronics, welding, and auto shop. With the exception of the upholstery class, I had both the education and the experience before taking the other classes. Still, the classes were better than working for nothing.

My instructors realized that I was not your average student and often left me to assist in teaching the classrooms. Without an adult peering over our shoulders, I got to teach things that they probably wouldn't have learned otherwise. For instance, it's hard to steal a car if you don't know how to hot-wire it. Piece of cake. Raise the hood, yank out a wire and connect it from the battery to the ignition coil. Put a screwdriver or knife across the solenoid and there you go.

Welding. Arc welding. Got a rod you're unfamiliar with and don't know how high to turn up the juice? Start low. If it sparks and sticks to the metal, turn up the current. Is the metal in the rod hard or soft? If it's hard, it's for welding hard metals like steel and iron. Soft might be for aluminum.

Electronics class really should have been called radio repair as that is what we mainly dealt in. The authorities were afraid we'd electrocute ourselves, or each other, if they gave us a television or anything else that ran on house current. So we mainly dealt with the 12 volt car radios that were periodically brought in.

In their defense, it was smart not to bring in tv sets. Those have high voltage transformers called flybacks. We're talking about tens of thousands of volts. Very dangerous. The televisions they make today run on much lower voltage and are, relatively safe.

One of the devices we used in class was an oscilloscope. That is a device that has a small television screen that shows different wave functions, types of waves, and their amplitude. It's kinda like looking at a moving picture of a flow of electricity. They were very expensive and there had been the added risk of somebody sticking a low current probe into a high voltage circuit (such as televisions had).

I was most attracted to auto shop. Well, in the beginning. You see, I had started driving when I was eight years old. I started racing cars when I was ten. For me, a Learner's permit was redundant as I could out-drive most adults and all of my instructors (I took driver's education in my last year of high school before being sent to reform school).

Not only did I race cars, I built them. I rebuilt my first engine at around twelve years of age. You know all of them lawnmowers that quit working when you ran over a rock? They quit because you broke or damaged a thing called a keeper key that aligns the flywheel with the crankshaft. It is softer metal and the rock caused the harder metals to cut into the softer metal of the key.

In the next chapter, we are going to look at more reasons for wanting to blow up the courthouse (as if I needed any). Reform school was just the tip of a much larger iceberg. Like the Titanic, this ship is going to sink. If any of this bores you, you can skip to the chapter (where I expose doctors for deliberately killing covid patients). I promise you, you won't be bored long.

Reasons for Blowing up Courthouse

I'm a sneaky little bastard. Just ask my wife. While I am explaining the things that my enemies will be trying to use against me, I am also exposing something that you either don't believe in or you never hear about. You were taught to respect authority and to uphold their law. But what do you do when you find out that they are the criminals and the law is wrong?

If I omitted this part, and I went straight to exposing doctors as ruthless murderers, you would have me committed and throw away the key. Nevermind that I can, and will, prove it. And do you yet realize why I have to tell you this part of the story?

Let's face it, in your world, you believe that the authorities would stop the doctors from doing their evil. I've already introduced you to some of those authorities. Still think they wouldn't let it happen? And I haven't even gotten to the bad guys yet!

When they let me out of reform school, I was placed in a foster home in Eugene, Oregon. About a year later, in June of 1971, I would graduate from Churchill High School. My foster parents liked me and had offered to let me stay there if I wished to pursue further education. It was an offer that, in hindsight, I should have accepted. But I didn't.

I had been in love with a girl from Dallas and had opted to return to my mother's house after being released by the juvenile authorities (upon graduation). I was looking forward to being with my girl.

A word of advice, if you want somebody to perform, especially a kid, you need to give him/her an incentive. In reform school, I had given up. Why? I had been working and going to school. Look where it got me. Why would I ever contemplate going to work or school if it was just going to cause me grief? It had to mean something, and it damned well should have meant something to the morons who decided to send me up the river...especially the goddamned Judge. Idiot.

I returned to Dallas, Oregon. In short order, I got myself engaged and was looking forward to growing old with a very special lady. I would return to work. And life was looking good again.

My fiancee was friends with a girl who lived in a very, very, very small town called PeeDee. Outside of a few homes and the sawmill, there wasn't much there. But that was enough.

According to my fiancee, her girlfriend had intimated that they needed workers at the mill. We drove out there one Saturday to talk to her girlfriend's father (who happened to be the foreman at the mill). He wasn't there, as I recall, but somebody told me to come back first thing Monday morning because that was the time that I would most likely get hired.

And so it was that I had gone out there. As soon as I pulled up, a man, presumably the foreman, called out to me and asked where the other guys were? Instinctively, I replied that I did not think they were going to make it. I later found out that they had been expecting three inmates to be released from jail for work release. None of the three made it. The good news was that I was hired on the spot. Oh happy days.

I loved working at the PeeDee mill. My job was pulling green chain. I was positioned at the head of the belt. That was where the cut up boards came out of the saw room. Often, the lumber would come out looking like a giant set of Pick-up Stix (sticks), and I'd have to jump up on the belt and untangle the mess. It was definitely a job for somebody young and in good shape. I was both.

One thing that I really liked about the job, besides the fact that it paid good, was that our boss was a wise old crow who cared about our health. He knew that most, if not all, of us went out drinking at night. In fact, we often went to a small tavern a few miles from the mill. Anyway, it was because of this knowledge that the owner, or whomever, had hired a cook and we always had a hot lunch. Otherwise, most drunks I knew did not get up in time to fix sandwiches or anything for lunch...not to mention going to the store.

Life was sweet. Things were going too perfect. Then I got busted one Saturday night for drinking. They took me to jail and the jailor asked me where I worked. I proudly boasted that I was working at the PeeDee Mill. Me and my big mouth.

Problem with my revelation was that I was only 17 years old at the time. To work in a mill, you were supposed to be 18. Oops. When they brought that up, I explained to them that I would be 18 when they released me Monday morning. Let that sink in.

On Monday I went back to the mill to go to work. I was promptly fired because the cops had called and told them I was only 17. The only time that the cops could have called was that morning and on that morning, I was 18. What kind of sick bastard destroys a man's life that way?

To say that the feud between me and the authorities escalated from that point on would be an understatement of Biblical proportions. I was sick and tired of Polk County authorities messing up my life. And when local lawyers refused to file a lawsuit against them for violating my Rights, I became determined to take them on myself, in my way, and on my time. Enough was enough.

There's an old adage that states that if you smack a dog with a stick enough times, he is going to bite you. To this day, I have no idea why Polk county assholes would think they were exempt. Of course, they all belonged to the same club, same gang, same synagogue, and thought they were invincible. They were soon to find out that just wasn't true.

Left without a job to provide me with some measure of stability, I partied more and more. I was at a party at a friend's house when we all ran out of cigarettes. Dallas was a small town where the favorite expression was "the streets roll up at night." It was pretty true. At three in the morning, even the taverns were closed. We needed cigarettes.

I seized upon that opportunity to enter the lion's den, so to speak, and we went to the only place in town that was open and had a cigarette machine. Yep, we went down to the police station. And yes, some of us were inebriated. And laughing and clowning around. It was a plan that worked perfectly. Huh?

To the cops, we were just a carload of dumbass drunks. We were certainly playing the part. Normally, drunks would try to appear incognito. Not us. We wanted the cops to chase us. Why?

Knowledge is power. Unbeknownst to our adversaries, we were sober. At least, I was. And I had formulated the plan, originally meant for a daytime "strike," but even more effective at night. In my pocket was a powder that makes people very sick without killing them. Somehow it fell on the floor. I'm not exactly sure how that happened. Perhaps a hole in my pocket. All I know is, by the time we did get home, it

46

had all fallen out.

As I slid into the driver's seat of my '66 Supersport, I knew I could outrun them, but chose not to. I just laughed as I watched the police single file their way out of the police station where we had just purchased our cigarettes. Their mindset was to arrest me, if not all of us, for being drunk in public. Ha ha.

I kept my eye on them as I slowly accelerated faster and faster away from them. At the end of Main street, I drove around the corner, killed my headlights and turned off onto a side road, then made another quick right and killed the engine. As we silently drifted to a stop, we could hear the police cars as they made the turn on Main street. When they did not see the taillights of my car, they assumed that I had floored it and raced away. We all laughed as they stomped their accelerator pedals to the floor and roared up the hill to try to catch us.

When we heard they had all gone, I restarted the car and drove a ways with the lights off. The route we took, took us to the edge of the football field at the local junior high. We shut the car down and got out to drink beer and smoke cigarettes.

When you have been harassed and abused to the extent that I had been, by the very people I was then taunting, you enjoy some measure of satisfaction in annoying the bastards. We reveled in that knowledge as none of us like the assholes running Dallas.

Eventually, we decided it was time to go back home. We took side streets and was actually back there for almost an hour before the cops showed up. The police were not happy but, then, they never were. They took me off to the side and wrote me out a citation for speeding. Allegedly, one of them had seen my taillights at the top of the hill (bullshit) and they had theorized that I must have been doing at least 60 in a 25mph zone. I tore the ticket up and told them to f@#k off.

They wrote another citation. It was for doing 80 in a 20mph zone. As the officer handed it to me, he warned me not to tear it up.

I was beyond mad. "F@#k you," I yelled as I ripped the paper in two.

Yes, I was shoved up against their car and handcuffed. Then I was driven down to the jail and booked in. To this day, I have no idea what charge, if any, they used for that. I was released the next day when my grandmother paid the five hundred dollar bail on the traffic citation. Just like there was no such charge as "Out of parental control," people did not go to jail for speeding. Likewise, such a citation does not require bail. But granny had paid it and I was released.

On the date listed on my Summons (a court order to show up in court), I walked into Judge Foster's courtroom. When he saw me, he stated that the prosecution was not ready to proceed and a court date would be rescheduled. After a couple of months, I got curious and went down to confront Foster about that new court date. When he told me that I had forfeited bail because I failed to appear, I went ballistic and grabbed a water pitcher and threw it at him. "F@#k you."

Foster had ducked down behind his desk and snuck into his chambers to hide. I threw a glass at the door. Then I stormed out of the courtroom. After that, according to rumors, the bastard started carrying a revolver. It mattered not as I would have thrown shit at him anyway. Sorry piece of crap.

Things would escalate from that point on. I won't bore you with all of the sordid details, but will try to gloss over the key parts. If you are interested in knowing more, I suggest you read my autobiography.

A lot of things were going on after that. The level of

corruption was escalating hourly. Things came to a head when I was arrested for first degree burglary for a crime that, not only did I not commit, no such crime had been committed.

My father had left to stay with his mommy again. My mother was struggling. I was unemployed and, sorry to say, too proud to go down and apply for foodstamps. Looking back, my mother should have let me starve, but she didn't.

My friends would come over to the house and they all called my mother "mom." It appeased her as she was a people person.

One night, a bunch of us were partying there when we decided to move the party from Dallas over to Salem; a distance of some fifteen miles. The reason was simple. My mother had to get up early in the morning to go to work and we did not want to keep her awake.

Three of us piled into a car driven by another friend. He had been dating a girl named Pam and was driving her car. As we neared the outskirts of town, Bill asked us if we were hungry. Well, hell yes. And so it was that we went to his house or, more specifically, to the house that he shared with Pam.

We were in hog heaven. There were three freezers full of meat that had recently been butchered. We grilled up some steaks. Of course, after eating, we all pretty much lost interest in going to Salem to party. At that point, Bill suggested that we take a couple boxes of the meat to my mother's house to help her out. And so it was.

Mother was elated. It was one less thing that she had to worry about.

Several days passed without incident. Then one night I was out partying and did not get home until 3am. I no sooner pulled up to my house when a Polk County (Dallas) deputy sheriff pulled up and asked me if I would be willing to go down to the sheriff's office to answer some questions. I had no idea what the hell was going on, but I knew I was drunk and even said so. The deputy said they didn't mind if I didn't.

And so it was that I climbed into his patrol car and went downtown. His name was Richard, commonly known as Dick. It fit him, as every time his partner left the room, the dick went into a rant about how I was guilty and he was going to see to it that I did a lot of time. You know it better as "good cop, bad cop."

I was not in the mood to be f@#ked with and returned fire. Frequently calling him a fat f@#k and anything else I could think of. It would be daylight before they would wrap it up.

The problem? As it turned out, Bill had not been living with Pam. She had been living with her parents and they had been out of town. I had no idea and acknowledged nothing. They also questioned me about Pam's checking account. Had I ever written any checks on it? No, of course not. And I gave them something like three pages of samples of my handwriting for comparison.

"Did I ever see Bill writing checks on her account?"

That one I answered truthfully. "Yes, I had." Pretty much every time that Pam got drunk, she would have him write, and sign, checks for her. No biggy.

Apparently it had been a biggy as Bill started writing checks without her permission or knowledge. I had no idea. But I had no reason to doubt it. Unlike me, Bill had an aversion to work.

The morning sun was up by the time deputy dog dropped me off at home and issued a stern warning: "I'm going to see that you go down...for a long time."

Knowing that I was innocent, I confidently replied "F@#k you, you fat bastard." And I went to bed. It had been a long night.

50

A few days later, I was pulled over and arrested for first degree burglary. Normally a person in my position would be granted bail on his own recognizance. That's just a lawyer word for be released on your word that you would show up in court. Though they all knew that I would show up, the request was denied. The Judge cited my juvenile record. That had nothing to do with flight risk or risk to the community. What's more, it was inadmissable. I had never failed to show.

To understand this refusal, you need to understand the criminal justice (sic) system. Most of the time, when they deny you bail, it is for a reason other than the two I just stated. And that was the case here. First off, they wanted to see if I would slip up and admit to the other inmates that I had knowingly stolen something. Secondly, they wanted to scare me into making a deal with them (in exchange for a reduced sentence). Third, they wanted to teach me a lesson for disrespecting them. But they did not know when to back off.

They refused to let my fiancee come in to see me. We were supposed to be getting married in a few short months and they wouldn't even let her letters in...except, of course, the one "Dear John" letter. Oh, that one they were glad to let in.

By the time that I received the Dear John letter, I already knew it was over. The jail was short-handed and they had asked me to be a trustee until they could find a replacement. The jailors all knew me, especially the head jailor, and they thought I was a nice enough guy. It was unheard of because trustees were only supposed to be inmates who had been found guilty and sentenced by the court. I was still awaiting the trial.

So how did I know that it was over between my fiancee and myself? Because I had looked out the window of the jail and saw her with another guy. He was driving her mom's new car and she was leaned up against him. Pretty obvious. I was crushed. That had been the last straw.

In her Dear John letter, she wrote that her parents were always telling her that I was no good; that I would always be no good. They based this on my having been sent to reform school and my history of going to jail. And you already know what a bunch of bullshit that was.

I was devastated; utterly crushed. It was so obvious that I was placed in isolation and put on suicide watch. I had no intention of committing suicide...at least not until I got some measure of revenge. But there was that god-awful radio and 'Sylvia's Mother' was playing thirty times a day. FYI, that was/is a very sad song wherein a fella had my plight. "And Sylvia's mother said, Sylvia's busy; too busy to come to the phone." Trust me, that's one experience that you never want to go through. Suicidal? Nope. Homicidal? No comment.

Ever hear that adage, "when it rains, it pours"? That is precisely what was about to take place. In Oregon, they could only hold you sixty days without taking you to trial. On my sixtieth day, they took me to the courtroom. I was shocked to see my (ex) fiancee and her mother in the courtroom. I listened as the Judge rattled off a bunch of legal mumbo-jumbo. It turns out that Pam had been sent by the police to gather incriminating evidence against me. Succinctly, she had gathered meat wrappers from mom's house.

From a legal standpoint, there was no way to tie those wrappers to me. Moreover, there was nobody willing, or able, to testify against me. The Judge dismissed the case based on Illegal Search and Seizure. I wasted no time jumping to my feet and objecting.

"You bastards have kept me in jail for two months for a goddamned crime that you knew I never did. My fiancee and her mother are in the courtroom so as to ascertain whether or not I am guilty. If you refuse to have a trial, then they will think I am guilty of something I am not guilty of."

The Judge banged his gavel and advised me to shut up and let my lawyer handle it. "That's not my lawyer," I screamed. That's your goddamned lawyer. If he were my lawyer, he would insist on a trial so I can prove my innocence. And I'm willing to wave whatever right I have to waive in order to get a goddamned trial."

The Judge did not even try to speak to me. He banged his gavel and declared, "case dismissed." Dirty sonsofbitches.

Clever bastards made sure there wasn't anything I could throw at the Judge. And they made sure that I couldn't run after him. Justice? Not yet, but I swore it would come soon.

As if I needed anymore reason to want to kill the bastards, I was about to discover even more. While I sat in jail, they served my poor mother with papers informing her that if she did not get rid of the cars around her house, they would fine her a hundred dollars a day and maybe even lock her up in jail. I had seventeen prized cars there. They were worth a lot of money and had been my primary source of income. Mom had to call the auto wreckers and they hauled my precious cars off for free. Payback, as they say, is a bitch.

Doctors are Killing Covid Patients

Before going further, I want to refresh your memory about what I said in the beginning. There are two types of really smart people. One is the memory-type of person and the other is the processor type. Remember?

It is important to remember that there are two types of people. Smart people anyway. But you also need to know how rare each is. About ten percent of the population consists of very intelligent people who can memorize stuff like crazy. It is phenomenal. Likewise, there is about ten percent of the people who have overblown processors. Most people are a mix and lie somewhere in between these two types.

How many times have you said that so and so was an idiot? A moron? Stupid? Dumb as a rock? Or whatever your favorite moniker happens to be? Most of us have. Some, more frequently than others.

Now let's take a look at why we are truly a world where the dumb are being led by the blind. Specifically, let's address antiquated and outdated textbooks. More succinctly, medical books.

Long before there were cures for many of the illnesses that we now know of, doctors were pretty limited on what they could and couldn't do for a patient. It was for this very reason that all medical care, past and present, says to make the patient as comfortable as possible. This is especially true of terminally ill people for whom the doctors have no remedial course of action for.

How ironic that the medical care is worse than the disease that they are trying to treat. Of course, in order to realize that, you need to have a processor and the vast majority of doctors are memory people...not just memory people, but memory people on the low end of the spectrum. What?

If you've ever had a course in First Aid, you were taught to make the victim as comfortable as possible. If in shock, make sure he/she is warm. You may remember these things, but you have lost sight of the very first, and most important, rule. Check the airway. Make sure the patient is breathing. Be sure that the airway is not obstructed in any way. And they even went so far as to admonish you to loosen their clothing so as to facilitate this end.

This is medicine that every single one of us has heard about and yet it is being ignored. Not only is it being ignored, it is being censored while doctors set about killing us. Don't think so? Look around moron. What do you see? Masks.

I suppose you want to know if doctors are killing people other than by forcing them to wear deadly masks? Let's look at some of them. Fauci is listed as a doctor...though my personal opinion of that idiot is that he is the last person who should have any pedigree in medicine.

And let's not forget about all of the doctors, and I do mean all of them, who know that wearing masks suffocates people. They may not be making us wear them by direct order, but they damned well are by not speaking up against masks.

Okay, so you can see where doctors may have something to do with suffocating old and sick people by inaction. You surely get that. But I'm here to tell you that they are doing even worse things to kill people---deliberately! There are exceptions, but eighty percent of the doctors are trying to kill their patients. Yes, deliberately!

At one time, one third of all covid deaths reported in Oregon were in the Veteran's Hospital in Portland, Oregon. Think that it was a coincidence, or do you honestly believe that military people have weaker immune systems? Wrong answer.

Covid 19, whether a real pandemic or not, is a respiratory disease. Any objections to that description? So what is it we have learned about the respiratory system? Don't obstruct the airway and make sure that the patient can breath. Basic First Aid. Common knowledge in the medical field. So why are doctors not adhering to this?

The short answer is that most doctors consider Covid 19 to be an incurable disease that often ends in fatalities. This is where their old school medical education kicks in. Sedate the patient and make sure they are comfortable. WTF!

When you have a respiratory disease, you have trouble breathing. Right? Right. Without question. So a doctor's first line of approach should be to assist a person in breathing. Correct? Correct. Why? Because the patient will suffocate if they do not.

At this juncture, I think you should look up suffocation. A person with a respiratory disease is, literally, suffocating. It is one of the most traumatic things that can happen to a human being, or any other life-form. The problem is, the majority of doctors are purposely suffocating patients. Ask them.

When a person is suffocating, it sends signals to the brain to do something to help alleviate that problem. Look it up. The brain then commands the heart to beat harder and faster. Simultaneously, the brain tells the lungs to breath deeper and harder and faster. Look it up. This is not crap that some brainiac is making up to scare the hell out of you. This is real-life what is going on.

Still don't see the problem? What happens when the

damned doctor sedates the patient? The drugs slow down the patient's pulse, slows down his respiration and makes his breathing more shallow. Shallow breathing does not allow oxygen to get deep inside the lungs (where it is needed the most). And the odds are exponentially high that the patient is going to succumb to the suffocation. And you can bet your ass that the damned doctors are going to claim that covid 19 killed another soldier. Or your mother, your father, your brother/sister, girlfriend/boyfriend, or significant other. Dead. Finito.

Still think doctors aren't deliberately killing people? Do you have any other explanation for why they are suffocating their patients? Yes, I know, you never gave it any thought. It is why you're a memory person and I'm a processor.

Think about all of those veterans. Many are getting paid pensions from their years of service. Most are getting paid disability and/or medical. All are costing the government in terms of treatments and drugs...not to mention the hospital stay. Give that some measure of thought.

Like it or not, if you are in charge of balancing the budget, your job entails trimming the fat. How does one do that? Do you take money away from the police departments? Fire? Schools? Or do you take it away from veterans by ending their lives? After all, they've already served their purpose. Right?

Your problem is that you do not believe that anybody would be so callous. Or, if you acknowledge that such people exist, you are of the belief that they are few and far between. And here I am accusing the entire medical profession? Have I lost my mind? You may think so now, but all of that is going to change before you get to the end of this book.

One of the problems inherent in trying to see the truth in something is that a person has biases, misperceptions, and pre-conceived beliefs, that cloud your vision. Whereas you see doctors as people who struggled through eight years of college so that they could help people, I see the reality. There are exceptions. But the things I speak of are of the majority.

There is no adage or fancy jingle to guide us and so I feel a need to create one. It might go something like this here: nurses nurse and doctors don't. What that means, generally speaking, is that nurses have compassion and genuinely care about their patients. They want to help make someone's life a little bit better.

Nursing is something that a doctor cannot afford to embrace. It is something that is ingrained into their heads during college. Nurses are generally women, and a woman's job is nurturing. Doctors, on the other hand, are generally men, and men have a tendency to take care of business and tune out the emotional side.

Doctors must, by the very nature of medicine, be able to shut down their emotions. If they could not do this, then they could not do things that hurt people. Nevermind that the treatment is going to effect a cure of some sort; it is hard to see someone going through pain. But doctors do it; don't they?

Another misconception that the majority of people have, as regards physicians, is that they are only doctors. Not true. Doctors must be, first and foremost, businessmen. If a doctor is not a business-oriented individual, he/she is not in business long. Even if a doctor has nothing but the best of intentions, that is to say, even if the doctor actually desires to help people to the best of his/her abilities, he/she knows that they must make money to sustain their practice. No way around that.

If you disbelieve any of that, go to a doctor's office and try to get in. Don't have medical insurance? Too bad. Don't have any money? So sad. It's a business. Never forget that.

I lived in Portland, Oregon, in the 1980s; when they first passed Mandatory Car Insurance. The City of Portland later announced that they had implemented a mandatory tow law that (mis)appropriated uninsured automobiles. The first week of that unjust law, they got on television and bragged that they had towed 742 cars that were not insured. I was outraged. Poor people often have to decide what bill not to pay, or they starve. Mandatory car insurance provided one more hardship for poor people that they really did not need.

How frigging warped do you have to be before you go on television and rejoice at causing 742 people misery? I promptly sat down and wrote a letter to the City Hall. In that letter, I warned them that I lived in my car and if they towed it, I was going to walk into City Hall and kill as many of the bastards as I could. I meant every single word. The fact that I am not, now, in prison shows that my car was not towed.

Their stated excuse for passing mandatory car insurance? According to the liars that did it, they did it because too many people were having uninsured accidents and it was costing the government too much money. What a crock of shit. Fact is, very few poor people were having accidents. For one thing, they were too broke to buy gas. No gas, no driving.

Secondly, almost all accidents were, and are, caused by people with money. They buy fancy SUVs or sports cars and think they are invincible. Crash. Uninsured? Perhaps. But almost always because some rich bastard was speeding and crashed into them.

Seriously, very few accidents involved uninsured motorists. The excuse was as lame as the assholes who passed it. And why would you force a poor family out of the relative safety of their car to live on the streets amongst common thugs? Are you frigging kidding me, you heartless bastards!

Did the law actually save the government money?

Absolutely not. In fact, just the opposite was true. You see, the government footed the bill for towing the cars. The government footed the bill for taking the poor people to jail. The government footed the bill for the now homeless street people. The government footed the bill for their trials, their lawyers, and their incarceration. I guarantee you, what little money the uninsured motorists were causing was a drop in the bucket compared to the ultimate price.

And the truly sad part about that whole charade was just the fact that, prior to the passing of the law, uninsured motorists weren't costing the government hardly a damned dime. Huh?

When there is an accident, it usually involves two vehicles. If one is uninsured, then the damages are assumed by the person with the insurance. And so it would have been the insurance companies and/or insured drivers that were footing the bill; not the damned government.

For the record, whether one car is insured, or both cars were insured, it was still going to cost the insurance companies. Greedy bastards.

In the first year of mandatory car insurance, most everyone I knew had their rates jacked up three times in just the first twelve months. And you're helpless because Uncle Sam will send the gestapo after you if you don't pay the blood-sucking demons.

I warned people that they would not stop there. It was only a matter of time before they got around to health insurance. And, if we continue to let the crooks in the insurance companies maintain those unconstitutional laws, we will soon have to get another job just to pay the insurance companies. Many people already do.

Not so long ago, I was getting $700 a month in social security. Medical insurance was $300. and my car insurance was well over a hundred. Every month. Tell me, douchbags, what was I supposed to live on?

Remember all of those Geico ads about saving you money? Lying bastards. Yes, I'm accusing Geico of fraud. Thieves. My insurance was over a hundred bucks with no tickets, no accidents, and never any DUIs. On top of that, I had driven eighteen wheelers for years. Safely. $113? Why?

I did the smart thing, after the representative told me they had given me every discount they had, I switched to Metromile. I could have gotten insurance at other places just as cheap, or cheaper than Metromile, but I liked the idea of only paying for miles driven. But even that isn't true.

Metromile charges you a flat monthly rate before tacking on milage. Convenient in that, if you did like I did and not drive very many miles, they could simply jack up your monthly rate. Even at the peak of their charges, Metromile was still less than half of what the bandits at Geico were charging me. Fifteen minutes can save you fifteen percent or more...but only if you switch to another company. F@#k Geico.

I remember that, in the years immediately preceding the passing of mandatory health insurance, major hospitals all over the country started building these huge monolithic structures. Salem (Oregon) Hospital had spent something like a million dollars building a new parking structure. As I recall, they immediately tore it down to build a new hospital. I say as I recall because there is a parking structure in the same vicinity and I want to see if the crooks admit to it or not.

Don't believe that organized crime would be involved in the medical profession? Are you really that ignorant? We all know the crooks run the insurance companies. We all know politicians are crooks. But somehow you think dealing with people's health is somehow exempt?

Success or failure is built upon the universal law of supply and demand. We all get sick and go to the doctors. All of us. It is about as big a business as any in existence. Do not, for even one instant, suppose that the big dogs do not have their corrupt fingers in the pot. How else would Salem Hospital, or any other institution, know to build superstructures before the Affordable Care Act was even a whisper? Please.

You know how much my medical costs were prior to affordable care? Exactly zero. I was on food stamps and medical came free. Now I'm on disability and/or social security. Very little comes out of my pocket because the government helps me. Without that help, my costs were around three hundred a month. And, no, the price did not go down. Fact is, the government pays for all of it.

Under the old regime, the government (my case workers) got to decide what medical treatments to approve. Under that premise, I went to the doctor sparingly. After they made it mandatory, all of that shit changed. Well, some of it.

Remember when they passed the law and insurance companies were trying to deny us care if we had pre-existing conditions? Imagine that...an insurance company actually having to pay for something!

So the government stopped that pick and choose bullshit. Now anybody can get insurance. Instead of cheap rates for healthy people, they charge ridiculous rates for everybody. And to top it off, the government foots the bill for a lot of it.

Look around you. How many giant buildings, skyscrapers, etc., are built and owned by insurance companies? How many sports arenas are owned by the insurance companies? Let's face it, those criminals are raking it in hand over fist. Let's see them deny it. And why hasn't the crooks in Congress stopped them from gouging us? Guess we know who's pocket all that ill-gotten gain goes into; don't we? Now even you know it.

One of the things about being a genius who sees things as they really are, is that I also see the solutions. In the case of mandatory car insurance, it should be immediately abolished. Since the government is footing the bill for locking up poor people and towing cars, the government should be getting that insurance payment. Only it shouldn't be an insurance payment, per se, it should be a payment paid to the Motor Vehicles Department every time you license your car. And that should be on a sliding scale (affordable) based on your income.

Think about the beauty of what I just said. Virtually every car on the road would be insured so long as it is currently licensed to be on the road. If it isn't licensed, then you might want to tow it. Every poor person on the planet, at least in civilized countries, can scrounge up a hundred dollars to license a car. So a sliding scale might look like 100-1,000. per year or whatever. My personal opinion is that, if you are a millionaire, you can afford to pay $10,000 or more.

Did you know that rich people don't even have to pay for car insurance? In Oregon, and other States, a person may post a $50,000 bond in lieu of paying an insurance company. This is yet another reason for tacking a fee on the car licensing. All cars. Make it fair; everybody pays.

As you can plainly see, money makes the world go 'round. Doctors are not exempt. Every time you go in to see them, there is a flat fee for the visit. Every time the doctor prescribes a pill or makes a referral to a specialist, there is a fee. And Lord help us if there happens to be shots or other procedures/surgeries. BTW, now you know why they made it so you have to have a referral to see a specialist. Besides getting more money, they get to refer you to their buddies.

It is important that you remember that medicine is a business. These stupid shots they are claiming protects you from Covid 19? Those are costing the taxpayer, on average, a thousand dollars a shot. Are you frigging kidding me? A thousand dollars? For what?

I better clarify something. When they first announced the shots, they told us that they were costing between 800 and 1200 per shot. After enough of us drew that to the public's attention, they had to downplay it. Now they claim those shots only cost about fifty dollars apiece. Bullshit. Even if the shot now cost fifty dollars to make, they still have to ship it. Have you forgotten the special containers and dry ice, etc?

And do not suppose that the doctors are injecting patients for free. It might be free to you but the government is paying for the cost of the medicine as well as shipping, handling, and injecting. Then there is waste disposal, follow-ups. And do not forget all of the millions that the government shelled out for research. Fifty dollars my ass.

Do you honestly think that booster shots are necessary? Well, actually, they are. You see, they cost a thousand bucks, too. Tell me, if you were in the medical field, wouldn't you want to be raking in a thousand bucks per person for every man, woman, and child, on the planet? Sure you would. But that doesn't mean we should be paying it.

Doctors are killing people simply because it is profitable for them to do so. Instead of charging a thousand dollars a shot, dying patients allow them to charge tens of thousands of dollars for ventilators, medicine, treatment, warehousing, and disposal. Yes, doctors charge for disposing of dead bodies.

And now we come to the really profitable part of the story. Doctors get paid tens of thousands of dollars just for saying that some sonofabitch died from covid. Yep. Remember what I said about incentive. As a businessman, there is no greater incentive then receiving a check from the United States government just for saying a patient died of covid. Hip-hip hooray!

I should like to take this opportunity to redirect you to the very first chapter. Do you remember the stats I posted that showed there was no spike in yearly, or even month to month, deaths? There was no spike in deaths. The only spike was in the number of lying-assed doctors who blamed covid for everything imaginable. Thirty thousand dollars is one hell of a lot of incentive. So Dr. Weissert certified people as crazy so he could make money. How many Dr. Weisserts are claiming covid deaths? More than you think; lots more.

And do not, for even one second, ever suppose that there are not doctors who deliberately kill their patients in order to get more money. If the truth were told, there are a lot of them.

While I cannot venture a guess as to how many doctors are killing their patients in order to get tens of thousands of dollars, I can estimate how many are making patients ill in order to make more money. I have a strong inclination to say that any doctor who prescribes a pill but, realistically, I know that I should be a trifle more conservative. Therefore, let's just say that any doctor who prescribes more than three medicines at a time or more than five in the course of a year. There are exceptions, as always, but not many.

Let's look at my medical history for the last five years.

Clues

The following is a chart of my blood pressure, pulse, and weight. I start with Dr. Brett Hayes, November 18, 2016, Dr. Mark Fischl, February 16, 2017, and go through to Dr. Fiorella Saavedra, December 17, 2020. This is data gleaned from the respective Doctor's notes.

Dr. Hayes-

11/18/2016:	182/112	86	285
12/15/2016:	150/96	92	287
01/19/2017:	154/92	77	283

Dr. Fischl-

02/16/2017:	113/81	85	273	
05/19/2017:	150/77	77	273	
08/21/2017:	140/81	69	276	
10/20.2017:	123/76	80	276	
12/07/2017:	136/78	70	277	
04/02/2018:	164/98	89	284	
07/03/2018:	128/79	88	286	
08/16/2018:	101/72	85	283	
09/22/2018:	123/72	80	278	
11/05/2018:	136/78	74	287	
04/11/2019:	138/73	72	289	respiration 22
07/16/2019:	132/73	84	281	

Author note:

I have been contacting various lawyers in an attempt to find one willing to sue Fischl. Subsequently, records have been changed and/or deleted. For instance, before contacting the lawyers, I had seen records for Brett Hayes all the way through 2016. Those have disappeared. Likewise, records for Dr. Fischl have disappeared. You will note that, according to the altered records, I only saw Fischl three times in 2019. However, I have, in my hot little hands, a lab report dated 10/03/2019. I am alleged to have seen Fischl on July 16, 2019. I then saw him on 10/17/2019 (two weeks after the lab) Labs do not take 3 months to complete. So what gives?

| 10/17/2019: | 138/88 | 64 | 283 |
| 01/31/2020: | 158/90 | 69 | 290 |

In December of 2019, I contracted Covid 19. It peaked on or about January 6, 2020. At that time, I lost all sense of taste and smell. Zero. Notta. Nothing. Zip. Despite my revelation to Fischl on January 31, that it was unlike anything I've ever had, he went ahead and tested me for the flu (influenza A & B). The test was negative. Duh. No test was available for covid unless I stated that I had come from China. You already know why (to blame the Chinese).

Or maybe you're a memory person who doesn't remember. You see, the United States wanted to make it look like the Chinese were responsible for creating covid 19. To do that, they ordered all doctors in the United States not to test for covid unless the person was Chinese or recently came from China. Why? Because the bug was manufactured in the United States and then spread to the rest of the world.

I have no idea when, or if, I got rid of the covid. My personal theory is that the virus is always present in all of us.

And I shall be explaining this in greater detail in an upcoming chapter. Meantime, I continued to be sick and actually got worse as time passed. On March 7, 2020, under threat from my siblings, I gave in and went to the hospital.

At the hospital, Dr. Lazeni Koulibali (an excellent physician) gave me a battery of tests and x-rays. He diagnosed me with Acute bronchitis and an upper respiratory infection (covid is an upper respiratory infection). He admonished me to see Fischl asap; no later than three days from then. March 7 had been a Saturday (night) and so I had to wait until March 9, Monday morning to go to Salem Clinic to see Fischl. But he refused to see me, and the receptionist told me they would call me with an appointment date.

After three more days, I opted to send Fischl an email message. He responded on March 12, 2020. I tried again and he responded on March 13, 2020. Somehow, between January 31 and March 12, 2020, Fischl had become a self-professed expert on Covid 19. Without ever testing me for that particular affliction, Fischl looked into his magic crystal ball and declared that I did not have covid 19. In his words, it had come and gone.

That's pretty amazing when you think about it. Nobody else in the entire world had any clue as to how covid 19 got around, how long it took to gestate, how long it lingers, nor pretty much anything else about it. Yet my doctor is an expert...even going so far as to say I did not even have it. And with no test!

But there had been a test; lots of tests. Dr. Koulibali had ordered a CBC. In that particular test, it was noted that my neutrophils were high and my lymphocytes were low. Both of these things are commonly found in Covid 19 patients. Considering the urgency expressed by Dr. Koulibali, I am thinking that he suspected as much, but had been ordered by the government not to test for covid. The best he could do was to urge me to see Fischl asap.

I, myself, have no exact date for when I got covid. I have no idea when, if ever, it went away. But I do know that it peaked on January 6, 2020/March 7, 2020, and that at least three of the symptoms persisted throughout the entire year.

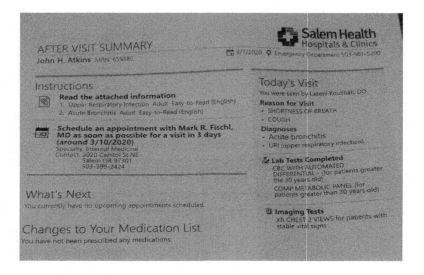

Doctor Fischl's messages perfectly reveal the extent to which his Munchausen's ran. He was always treating me for things I did not have and not treating me for the things I did have. Most importantly, he had not heeded a word I said and considered me to be lower than the slime on a slug's belly.

When Fischl refused to see me on March 9, and no appointment was forthcoming, I decided to try to effect a cure or, at the very least, make it so I could breath again. I settled on a drug called Gentamicin because it would treat the covid 19 long symptoms, particularly the respiratory infection, and definitely would help with the bronchitis. Specifically, I wanted it in liquid form so I could inhale it. Unbeknownst to me, Gentamicin actually comes in a nebulizer. That is something which Fischl, an internal medicine specialist, would have known. Instead of prescribing the medicine for me, Fischl took my messages to his bosses at Salem Clinic and they jointly decided not to save my life. On or about March 17, 2020, They sent me a certified letter from them informing me that Fischl would not be seeing me anymore.

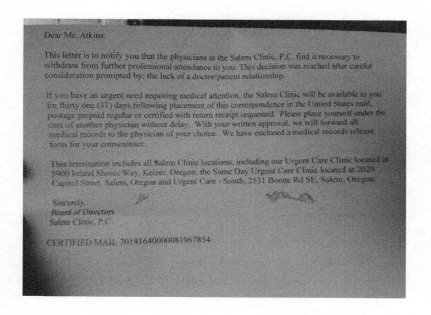

Dear Mr. Atkins:

This letter is to notify you that the physicians at the Salem Clinic, P.C. find it necessary to withdraw from further professional attendance to you. This decision was reached after careful consideration prompted by: the lack of a doctor/patient relationship.

If you have an urgent need requiring medical attention, the Salem Clinic will be available to you for thirty one (31) days following placement of this correspondence in the United States mail, postage prepaid regular or certified with return receipt requested. Please place yourself under the care of another physician without delay. With your written approval, we will forward all medical records to the physician of your choice. We have enclosed a medical records release form for your convenience.

This termination includes all Salem Clinic locations, including our Urgent Care Clinic located at 5900 Inland Shores Way, Keizer, Oregon, the Same Day Urgent Care Clinic located at 2020 Capitol Street, Salem, Oregon and Urgent Care - South, 2531 Boone Rd SE, Salem, Oregon.

Sincerely,
Board of Directors
Salem Clinic, P.C.

CERTIFIED MAIL 70191640000081967854

Moreover, I was not to come into any of Salem Clinic's facilities. I received that letter some time in the first half of April.

I realize that you do not think anything about the timing of that decision/letter, so I shall enlighten you. At that time, doctors were not seeing new patients. Within a couple of weeks, early April, everything was shutting down and doctors were not even seeing their old patients. By the time I got the letter, there were no new doctors available to me.

I believe that Fischl and his cronies were completely disregarding the medical diagnosis regarding bronchitis from Salem Hospital and solely concentrating on covid. So I'm going to address that issue right now.

Under both State and Federal law, if a patient has a life-threatening disease, particularly one in which there is no known cure, the patient has the absolute right to try any medicine or procedure that the patient believes may save his life. Period. Wherefore Fischl, and his cronies at Salem Clinic violated my Constitutional Rights, did so unconscionably and maliciously, and did cause me permanent and substantial damage, with complete disregard for my pain and suffering. Remember, they could not tell me that I did not have covid without conducting a test. And this was in spite of tests that clearly showed I could have had it. Still want to insist doctors were not trying to kill people deliberately?

Bearing in mind that Fischl saw me on January 31, 2020, and he did not prescribe anything, and he fired me in March, that left me without any medical attention for almost all of 2020, I suffered for a whole year needlessly. On December 17, 2020, I finally got a new doctor, a Physician's assistant by the name of Fiorella Saavedra. Let's resume with the clues.

Dr. Fiorella Saavedra:

12/17/2020:	193/105	no pulse listed	297lbs
01/06/2021:	144/79	no pulse listed	286lbs
04/27/2021:	136/80	no pulse listed	290lbs

That 193 over 105 had happened on a good day. By the time I saw Fio (rella), I had been without any medication, whatsoever, for months (thank you , Mr. Fischl). My normal blood pressure had persisted around 205 over 110 for the better part of four months. So, yes, 193/105 was good. Not!

Sometime in early June, 2021, my poop turned white. Yes, absolutely white. In addition, it didn't smell like regular poo; it was horrid, rancid, acrid, nasty smelling. If you ever have the pleasure of smelling that smell, you'll never complain about your poop fragrance ever again. Good God!

At first, I had no clue as to what was causing it. I did as I always did (post Fischl) and tried to self-diagnose. Typically, pale stool is caused by a lack of bile in your intestines. But what caused the lack of bile?

Medical literature provided many answers to the question of reduced bile. Diet could contribute to it. A lack of exercise, under the right conditions, could do it. Mainly, it could be caused by organ failure or some kind of bacterial infection or parasite. I was interested.

I quietly contemplated the multitude of data available to me, along with what I knew my symptoms to be, and concluded that I could have a bacterial infection. And I was positive that I had some kind of parasite.

Because I frequently hung out by a small stagnant water pond, I felt reasonably sure that whatever I had, came from there. There was black water, algae, and no life beyond a few bullfrogs. No birds. No bugs. It was, and is, eery.

Every day, I could feel "bugs" gnawing away at my innards. I was convinced that I had to have Giardia. I called Fio and tried to schedule an appointment. A Dr. Peter Bodmer got on the phone and we had a teleconference. He determined that it was serious enough to send me to get a cat scan.

It took about a week to get in, have the test, and then get

73

the results of the scan. All of my organs looked good. Although I had renal cysts (on the kidneys), they were nothing to be concerned about. In other words, whatever was causing the loss of bile was not an organ failure. That put me one step closer to my diagnosis of Giardia.

I thanked the person who called me to give me the results of the test, but what about the pale stool? Instead of scheduling more tests, or simply making an appointment, the person stated that I needed to talk to a doctor. Then they asked when I was seeing one? I informed him I was seeing my Urologist in two weeks. "Oh good," he said gleefully. "You can speak to him about it."

All of my life I have been passive. I really should learn to be more assertive. Problem is, there is a fine line between assertive and aggressive. And my experience taught me that any show of assertion would be interpreted as aggression. Best just to wait.

As expected, the urologist didn't know a damned thing about pale stool. I needed to see my primary care doctor. Do you think? I put in another phone call to Fio's office. And an appointment was scheduled for July 29, 2021.

Unlike Fischl, Fio listened. Even though we were at loggerheads of sorts in our respective diagnostics, she relented and tested me for the Giardia. Her opinion was that it might be a really rare bug that was making the rounds. I do not remember the name but it started with an m. But she did not stop there and ordered a battery of tests.

We were both wrong. The tests revealed that I had h. pylori (a bacterial infection) and blastocysts (parasites). For the record, my blood pressure had been 181 over 81 and my weight had dropped to 279.

According to the research I have done, it is safe to assume that I had both the infection and the parasites for several years. It is bore out by the rise and fall of my weight. It is also evidenced by other symptoms. Pulse, blood pressure, and pain. And substantiated by the extent of the damages it has done to me.

On July 16, 2019, Fischl had ordered x-rays to try to ascertain where my chronic back pain was originating from. On October 17, 2019, I told Fischl that I was drinking cranberry juice and a sports type drink called Body Armor. I revealed that the drinks were making my back feel much better. Though he did not write it down, he had told me: "placebo effect."

Think about that for a minute. Had my doctor took me at my word, instead of being an arrogant ass, he would have been thinking, "what causes back pain and can be alleviated by drinking cranberry juice?"

The answer, in case you haven't figured it out, is a bacterial infection. Had Fischl done his job instead of looking for ways to belittle me, he would have ordered up the very tests that Fiorella would order more than a whole year later. And I would not have suffered so long or as badly. Moreover, the damages done by any of the bugs would have been less severe.

Another symptom of h. pylori is that it causes nerve damage. By the time that I saw Fischl in the second half of 2019, I had already told him about the loss of feeling in the fronts of my lower legs and in my toes. Beyond tapping my knees with a rubber mallet and getting mad because I was not responding, he did nothing. Now I do not know about your neck of the woods but, where I come from, any nerve damage is cause for concern.

So far, you might be of the opinion that Fischl was just negligent. In the next chapter, I am going to prove to you that Fischl was deliberately, wantonly, and unconscionably, causing me substantial bodily harm. And to make things worse, he was trying to portray me as crazy. I shall let the records speak for themselves.

"Lack of doctor/patient relationship."

If you ever want to know what abusers do when they can no longer control you, ask an abused woman. He/she will kick you to the curb. And so it was that Fischl went to his superiors and cited a lack of doctor/patient relationship. That was the statement they published in their letter to me, dated March 17, 2020, when they fired me. Huge mistake. They should have fired Fischl.

In the preceding chapter, I revealed clues that clearly show that Fischl was willfully negligent by refusing to listen to me and criminally culpable for wrongly prescribing medication I did not need. In this chapter, we are going to discuss why it wasn't simple negligence but actual criminal intent to cause bodily harm. Let's start with the very first time that I met him.

On February 16, 2017, I met Fischl for the very first time. He seemed amicable enough, a little stiff, but amicable nonetheless. Little did I suspect that he was stabbing me in the back right from day one.

If you look at the lists (preceding chapter) I made regarding dates and vital signs, you will note that, the first time I met Fischl, my blood pressure was 113/81, my pulse was 85, and my weight was 273 pounds. Compare that to my vitals for January 19, 2017 (less than a month earlier). B.p. 154/92, pulse 77, and 283lbs.

That had been a huge shift in little over three weeks. As a doctor, I would have been concerned about such huge moves.

Fischl does appear to address this by having some tests done. The tests that he does order were not tests to try to determine the cause of the swings, rather, he seeks to assess the damages done so far. Why? Because he already knew what caused it. So he orders a test to see if my magnesium level is too low. He also orders tests to try to determine if my electrolytes have dropped and if my potassium was too low. Let's see if I can clarify this.

Allegedly, I saw Brett Hayes for the last time on January 19, 2017. On that date, allegedly, Hayes had me on a water pill and added a second. These were Chlorthalidone, and spironolactone. Two water pills. Got it?

Why did I state allegedly? Because I simply do not remember seeing Dr. Hayes on that date. Taking into account the way in which records seemed to be getting altered, and the ease one would have in altering such records, I suspect that Fischl, and not Hayes, may have switched them. Keep in mind that I have not, as yet, proven that to be the case; it is only a suspicion. Fischl should be regarded as innocent until proven guilty.

The question thus arises, why would I suspect Fischl? One reason is because of the way in which Fischl sought to destroy my health. Deliberately. Probably the most damning reason is simply how fast Dr. Hayes had disappeared. No warning. No advanced notice. No goodbyes. Nothing. It struck me odd. But then I realized that Fischl could not do the illegal things he does without his bosses being part of the scheme. So my question is this: did Hayes quit because he did not want to be part of any scheme wherein pills were prescribed to increase profits by purposely making the patient ill?

What do water pills do? They make you pee. They make you pee a lot. Fischl was always talking about my frequent urination and trying to blame it on old age or my prostate or whatever. Fact is, it was the water pills. And that was his intent.

You don't get it, do you? Old people my age generally have two things going on. Let me rephrase that, old men my age. First, there is the enlarged prostate. It is a fact of life that a man's prostate grows bigger with age. It is a normal rite of passage, so to speak. It is criminal for a doctor to treat it as "abnormal" when it is really normal. Of course, we have to ask, how would they even know it was enlarged if they had never known me when it was "normal"? To make matters worse, the prostate could be normal and the doctor can still claim enlarged.

The second problem inherent in old people is dehydration. It is a fact of life that, as we grow older, we lose our sense of thirst. What that means is, as we grow older, we tend to drink less water. That means that old people are suffering from dehydration. Look that up. D-e-h-y-d-r-a-t-i-o-n.

In his after visit summary, Dr. Hayes noted that I was being diagnosed with two things. Hypertension (high blood pressure) and an enlarged prostate. As I said, an enlarged prostate is normal for old men. Therefore, Dr. Hayes did not prescribe anything for that.

In his after visit summary some three weeks after Hayes', Fischl notes that I'm now diagnosed with high blood pressure, enlarged prostate, urinary frequency, and hypokalemia. While Fischl does cut one of the water pills in half, he adds a rather vicious one: Flomax (Tamsulosin). Think about it a minute.

In hypokalemia, the level of potassium in blood is too low. A low potassium level has many causes but usually results from vomiting, diarrhea, adrenal gland disorders, or use of diuretics. A low potassium level can make muscles feel weak, cramp, twitch, or even become paralyzed, and abnormal heart rhythms may develop.

79

Fischl knew for an absolute fact that the (diuretics) two water pills were causing me substantial harm. He orders tests to see to what extent. He sees that I am heading towards a serious potassium deficiency. He prescribes a potassium supplement and reduces one of the water pills to half dosage. But then he makes it even worse by prescribing Flomax. Why?

Flomax is a pill that relaxes the muscles in the prostate so that you can pee more easily. But it also relaxes the muscles in the bladder to allow a more complete release of water. So, in addition to frequent urination, now I'm peeing more at a time which, as Fischl knows, will lead to all kinds of things that are commonly associated with the dehydration. Primarily, it affects the kidneys and depletes things like magnesium and potassium.

For people with kidney disease: Chlorthalidone can make your kidney problems worse. Talk with your doctor about whether taking this drug is safe for you. For people with liver disease: Chlorthalidone can cause changes in your fluid and electrolyte levels. This may even lead to coma.

Fischl was obviously concerned about my kidneys being damaged but, instead of stopping the Chlorthalidone, he just cuts the dosage in half. Chlorthalidone produces slightly greater reductions in blood pressure compared with hydrochlorothiazide (HCTZ), but it is associated with greater declines in serum potassium levels.

Back in the 1970s, I had been hospitalized with hepatitis. That is a serious affliction of the liver that leaves permanent damage. Chlorthalidone should never have been prescribed in the first place.

We know for an absolute fact that Fischl is aware that the pills are causing me substantial harm. Dehydration can cause an increase in your pulse rate (such as the 85 in my file). And it causes weight loss. In this case, ten pounds in three weeks. Oh-oh. Two very important clues that I was dehydrated and Fischl prescribes a third water pill?

Bear in mind that, on the day that I first saw Fischl, my blood pressure was at an all-time low. 113/81 was a dream. A normal doctor would have been concerned about my blood pressure continuing on the rapid downward spiral. It was 154/92 just three weeks earlier. The prudent thing would have been to reduce, or even eliminate, one of the pills and wait another month to see how my body was going to adjust.

It is important that you keep this in mind because the Flomax was a potential death sentence. My blood pressure was dropping and he puts me on another pill that dehydrates and drives up blood pressure. Holy cow. It is a wonder I survived. But maybe that had been his plan. He felt he could blame it on Hayes. But he was wrong.

Then Fischl did something totally unwarranted and further put my health at risk: he scheduled me an appointment for three months away. Three months. My blood pressure was dropping. My pulse was high. My weight was decreasing. And he wants to wait three months to see if I was still alive?

It was a calculated risk because Fischl knew the Flomax would dehydrate me and drive up my blood pressure. Dehydration can lead to an increase in blood pressure due to the action of a hormone called vasopressin. Vasopressin is secreted when there's a high amount of solutes (or sodium level) in your blood, or when your blood volume is low. Both of these things can happen when you lose too much fluid. In response, when you're dehydrated, your kidneys reabsorb water as opposed to passing it in urine. High concentrations of vasopressin can also cause your blood vessels to constrict. This can lead to an increase in blood pressure.

When Fischl purposely set out to dehydrate me, he knew

that my blood pressure would rise instead of falling. Whereas I could die if my blood pressure dropped too low, he was reasonably certain I would survive an increase in blood pressure. So he opted not to see me for three months.

Knowing what I just told you, what do you think my vitals were the next time I saw Fischl on May 19, 2017? Yep. My bp had shot up to 150/77. It was a moral certainty. Predictable. And it happened.

Fischl's acts went way beyond reckless endangerment. His acts/inaction were causing me to be sick. Not just in 2017, when we first met, but for the entire three years that he was my physician. He was narrow-minded and short-sighted. He disregarded the things that I was suffering from and concentrated on making money by making me ill.

Let's see if we can make any sense out of my medical history; particularly the drugs.

Dr. Hayes-
11/18/2016:   182/112   86   285
meds:
1. Amlodipine increased from 5mg to 10mg
2. Start taking Chlorthalidone 25mg
3. Start Finasteride 5mg
4. Stop taking hydrochlorothiazide 25mg
5. Stop taking Tamsulosin .4mg
Diagnosis:
1. Essential (primary) hypertension
2. BPH (benign prostatic hyperplasia)
3. Need for influenza vaccine

*Author:

Dr. Hayes must have realized that I was suffering from

dehydration as he reduces one water pill and discontinues the worst one (Tamsulosin). The result was that my bp dropped.

12/15/2016:   150/96   92   287
meds:
1. Amlodipine 10mg
2. Chlorthalidone increased to 100mg
3. Finasteride 5mg
Diagnosis:
1. Essential (primary) hypertension

*Not sure why he increased the water pill. Maybe it was his way of trying to see if dehydration was really a problem. At any rate, we can predict that my bp was going to rise.

01/19/2017:   154/92   77   283
meds:
1. Amlodipine 10mg
2. Chlorothalidone 100mg
3. Finasteride 5mg
4. Start taking Spironolactone 25mg
5. Taladafil (Cialis) 2.5mg
Diagnosis:
1. Essential (primary) hypertension
2. Enlarged prostate w/o Luts (lower urinary tract symptoms)

* Not sure why Hayes added another water pill, Spironolactone. Spironolactone is commonly known as a potassium-sparing diuretic, which means in exchange for relieving the body of sodium and water, it makes the body retain potassium. This is how spironolactone works to protect the heart and lower blood pressure.

One test result showed that I had twice the triglyceride level that would be considered normal. The most common causes of high triglycerides are obesity and poorly controlled diabetes. If you are overweight and are not active, you may have high triglycerides, especially if you eat a lot of carbohydrate or sugary foods or drink a lot of alcohol.

Sugary food and drinks, saturated fats, refined grains, alcohol, and high-calorie foods can all lead to high levels of triglycerides. Guilty.

1. Refined Grains and Starchy Foods
2. Enriched or bleached white bread, wheat bread, or pasta.
3. Sugary cereals.
4. Instant rice.
5. Bagels.
6. Pizza.
7. Pastries, pies, cookies, and cakes.

Lord, I'm a sinner. I daily feasted on all of those things, excepting bagels. Maybe Hayes thought he could drive those things out of my system by frequent urination. One thing is for certain, the Spironolactone apparently drove out the deadly salt I was consuming in mass.

Dr. Fischl-

02/16/2017:   113/81   85   273
meds:
1. Amlodipine 10mg
2. Chlorothalidone 100mg (reduced to 50mg)
3. Finasteride 5mg
4. Spironolactone 25mg
5. Taladifil 2.5mg

6. Start taking Tamsulosin .4mg
7. Start taking Potassium Chloride ER 20 meq
Diagnosis:
1. Essential (primary) hypertension
2. urinary frequency
3. Enlarged prostate w/o luts
4. hypokalemia

* As already stated, my blood pressure was excellent. It is an absolute mystery why Fischl would intercede a process that was working. But he does. The Chlorthalidone is a prescription drug used to treat high blood pressure (hypertension). Lowering high blood pressure helps prevent strokes, heart attacks, and kidney problems. It is also used to reduce extra salt and water in the body caused by conditions such as heart failure, liver disease, and kidney disease.

We can say the same thing for the potassium-sparing Spironolactone. But it is beyond medical science why in the world Fischl prescribed as harsh a water pill as Tamsulosin. Tamsulosin helps reduce the symptoms of an enlarged prostate gland by relaxing the muscles in the bladder and prostate so you can pee more easily. It is neither potassium-sparing nor salt reducing. This is all the more shocking when you consider that the Finasteride was already being used for the enlarged prostate. We can easily predict that the additional water pill (Tamsulosin) is going to elevate my blood pressure.

05/19/2017:   150/77   77   273
meds:
1. Amlodipine 10mg
2. Chlorthalidone 50mg
3. Finasteride 5mg
4. Start taking Irbesartan 75mg

5. Tamsulosin .4mg
6. Spironolactone 25mg
7. XR Post Void test

*note: XR post void residual test to measure bladder capacity. Suspicion caused by water pills. Three months after we began our journey, the asshole has me on six damned pills and looking to prescribe more. Wtf!

Diagnosis:
1. urinary frequency
2. Essential (primary) hypertension

08/21/2017:   140/81   69   276
meds:
1. Amlodipine 10mg
2. Chlorthalidone 50mg
3. Finasteride 5mg
4. Irbesartan (increase to 150mg from 75mg)
5. Spironolactone 25mg
6. Tadalafil (Cialis) 2.5mg
7. Tamsulosin (Flomax) .4mg
Diagnosis:
1. Hypokalemia (primary)
2. Essential (primary) hypertension
3. Urinary frequency
4. Elevated Lipids
5. Need for hepatitis C screening test

* By this time, it was clear that Fischl was all about making money. When I saw him for the first time, my blood pressure was fine. I was doing good. But if Fischl leaves everything alone, there is no money in it for him. How insane that he had

me on six goddamned pills (I didn't include the Cialis because I had asked for that one but never took it).

It was a self-fulfilling prophecy wherein he gets to add ailments to my list. More ailments means more money for him. Instead of hypertension, I then had frequent urination from the water pills, Hypokalemia (low potassium) from the water pills, elevated lipids from the water pills, and an increased risk of getting hepatitis (a liver problem) which is also a result of the water pills (Chlorthalidone in particular).

10/20.2017:   123/76   80   276
meds:
1. Amlodipine 10mg
2. Chlorthalidone 50mg
3. Finasteride 5mg
4. Irbesartan (decrease to 75mg from 150mg)
5. Spironolactone 25mg
6. Stop taking Tadalafil (Cialis) 2.5mg
7. Tamsulosin (Flomax) .4mg
Diagnosis:
1. Need for influenza vaccination
2. Screen for colon cancer
3. Essential (primary) hypertension

* Six pills. Time to add procedures in order to make more money. Flu shot. Screen for colon cancer. More money. Referral to friend.

12/07/2017:   136/78   70   277
meds:
1. Amlodipine 5mg (decreased from 10mg)
2. Chlorthalidone 50mg

3. Finasteride 5mg
4. Irbesartan (increase from 75mg to 150mg)
5. Spironolactone 25mg
6. Tamsulosin (Flomax) .4mg
Diagnosis:
1. BPH
2. Essential (primary) hypertension
3. Lumbar strain, initial encounter
4. Hypokalemia

* Here he diagnoses me with a lumbar strain. It was a misdiagnosis founded on bad science. The water pills had dehydrated me to the point that my kidneys ached. It is noteworthy that Fischl makes the diagnosis by looking into his infamous crystal ball. An x-ray would have been in order.

04/02/2018:   164/98   89   284
meds:
1. Amlodipine 5mg
2. Chlorthalidone 50mg
3. Finasteride 5mg
4. Irbesartan (increase from 150mg to 300mg)
5. Spironolactone 25mg
6. Tamsulosin (Flomax) .4mg
Diagnosis:
1. Hypokalemia
2. Essential (primary) hypertension
3. BPH

* Look at my pulse. It is a key indicator that I was suffering from dehydration. Ditto for my high blood pressure.

07/03/2018:   128/79   88   286

meds:
1. Amlodipine 5mg (if bp drops below 115/70, stop taking)
2. Chlorthalidone 50mg
3. Finasteride 5mg
4. Irbesartan 300mg
5. Spironolactone 25mg
6. Tamsulosin (Flomax) .4mg
Diagnosis:
1. BPH
2. Essential (primary) hypertension
3. Snoring
4. Witnessed apneic spells

* Fischl was determined to keep me on six pills. More money. By now, I was experiencing apneic spells caused by, you guessed it, dehydration.

08/16/2018:   101/72   85   283
meds:
1. Stop taking Amlodipine 5mg
2. Chlorthalidone 25mg (reduced from 50mg)
3. Finasteride 5mg
4. Irbesartan 300mg
5. Spironolactone 25mg
6. Tamsulosin (Flomax) .4mg
7. Start taking Sertraline (Zoloft) 100mg
Diagnosis:
1. Essential (primary) hypertension
2. Hypokalemia
3. Generalized Anxiety disorder

* Here he prescribes Sertraline for the anxiety disorder. My bp was dropping so he stopped one of the bp pills. Problem

was, Sertraline causes a drastic drop in blood pressure. When my blood pressure dropped so low that I passed out, I stopped the Sertraline. I also went online and accused him of trying to kill me. As a specialist in internal medicine, Fischl knew the Sertraline would greatly reduce my blood pressure. He also knew that the drugs and/or dehydration could have been causing my depression/anxiety. That anxiety would ultimately go on to full-blown panic attacks.

09/22/2018:   123/72   80   278
meds:
1. Finasteride 5mg
2. Irbesartan 300mg
3. Spironolactone 25mg
4. Tamsulosin (Flomax) .4mg
5. Stop taking Chlorthalidone 25mg
6. Start taking Sertraline 50mg if bp is okay (was too low)
Diagnosis:
1. Need for influenza vaccination
2. Hypokalemia
3. Essential (primary) hypertension

* Fischl had me reduce the dosage of sertraline to half when he first prescribed it. Here, he is claiming that he is now reducing it. Excuse me doc, but it isn't reducing when you have me taking the same amount that caused me trouble to begin with. I still got dizzy and passed out. A check on my bp revealed that it was dangerously low, something along the lines of 60/40. Thanks, but no thanks. I was down to five pills a day instead of seven.

It is noteworthy that Fischl finally realizes that my high pulse rate and apneia is due to dehydration. He stops one of the three water pills.

11/05/2018:   136/78   74   287
meds:
1. Finasteride 5mg
2. Irbesartan 300mg
3. Spironolactone 25mg
4. Tamsulosin (Flomax) .4mg
5. Triamcinolone .1% cream
6. Stop Sertraline
Diagnosis:
unchanged/not given

*Note:
    On 3/21/2019, I saw Robyn Edwards (behaviorist) per Fischl referral. Superficial replacement for Sertraline. More money.

04/11/2019:   138/73   72   289 respiration 22
meds:
1. Finasteride 5mg
2. Irbesartan 300mg
3. Spironolactone 25mg
4. Stop taking Tamsulosin (Flomax) .4mg
5. Stop taking Triamcinolone .1% cream
6. Was given Pneumococcal vaccine, 13 valent
Diagnosis:
1. Need for pneumococcal vaccination
2. Essential (primary) hypertension
3. BPH
4. Witnessed apneic spells
5. Cough
6. Hypokalemia
7. urinary frequency

91

* It had been more than two years since I first started seeing Fischl. In that time, he destroyed the ideal 113/80 bp I had and replaced it with higher numbers. He put me on so many water pills that my dehydrated state worsened and caused my kidneys to start malfunctioning (chronic back ache), apneic spells, low potassium, urinary frequency, and a cough (later attributed to h. pylori, high bp, and parasites.

At long last, he finally stopped that god-awful Tamsulosin. It was the first time, to my knowledge, that he actually noted my increased respiration.

07/16/2019:   132/73   84   281
meds:
1. Irbesartan 300mg
2. Spironolactone 25mg
3. Start taking Fexofenadine 180mg (allergy pill)
4. Start taking Meloxicam 15mg (NSAID pain reliever used to treat arthritis such as in my spine)
5. Stop taking Finasteride
Diagnosis:
1. Essential (primary) hypertension
2. Generalized anxiety disorder
3. Witnessed apneic spells
4. Hypokalemia
5. Chronic bilateral low back pain w/o sciatica

*Note:
        I do not recall ever taking Meloxicam. This only materialized once I contacted a lawyer about suing Fischl for malpractice in ignoring my symptoms and especially for ignoring my revelation about the cranberry juice and Body Armor making my back pain go away. In his words: "placebo effect."

This was an important clue because cranberry juice does not fix backs or make them feel better. It does, however, work to fight off bacterial infections such as the h. pylori I was suffering from.

It is particularly noteworthy that every single one of the diagnoses listed are symptoms associated with dehydration and/or h. pylori. Keep in mind that Dr. Hayes had me down to one problem, hypertension. Under Fischl, that list grew exponentially.

10/17/2019:   138/88   64   283
meds:
1. Irbesartan 300mg
2. Spironolactone 25mg
3. Stop taking Fexofenadine 180mg
4. Stop taking Meloxicam 15mg
Discussion:
1. "Hypertension blood pressure well controlled. Labs look normal."
2. BPH symptoms, still with urinary frequency and nocturia
3. Snoring and probable sleep apnea
4. Significant back pain no radicular symptoms.

*Note:
There would have been only two reasons for Fischl to stop the allergy and the anti-inflammatory (erroneously called a pain pill). Either the drugs did not work or the drugs were causing more damages. My money is on both (assuming that he ever gave me Meloxicam). It is also at this point that Fischl acknowledges that I was living in my car. He mentions that I was using the cranberry/Body Armor cocktail and no longer needed an anti-inflammatory.

This was a very important clue as to what was really going

93

on and Fischl disregards it by calling it "placebo effect." In the entire history of medicine, no bad back was ever cured by a fruit cocktail; but UTIs and kidney infections were. How ironic that he keeps listing hypokalemia and renal failure but does not connect the obvious dots. Accident? Negligence? No way. The man had poured so many diuretics into me in order to cause renal failure. Once he achieved some measure of success in that area, he immediately began cutting back the water pills. That's how Munchausen's works. In the span of a few months, I had gone from six pills a day to two. In other words, I was getting better because he was taking away the damned pills that he had given to me to make me sick in the first damned place!

After dropping virtually all of the bad meds he had been wrongly prescribing all those years, look at what our hero notes: "Hypertension blood pressure well controlled. Labs look normal." My blood pressure was anything but well-controlled. And he notes that labs appear normal (now that I was off the drugs he gave me to make me sick). Still think he's innocent?

01/31/2020:   158/90   69   290
meds:
1. Irbesartan 300mg
2. Spironolactone 25mg
Diagnosed:
1. Fever
2. cough
3. Tested for influenza A & B. negative.

*Note:
I had gotten covid 19 in December of 2019. It peaked on or about January 6, 2020. At that time I lost all sense of taste

and smell. I also lost the ability to breath and had a bad cough. Fischl knew this on January 31, but refuses to test for either the Covid or the after effects of covid.

Covid 19 is a respiratory disease that usually results in one of two respiratory problems. The worst of these is pneumonia. This is what killed the people in Wuhan and alerted the authorities to the problem. Most victims that are alleged to have died of covid, actually succumbed to pneumonia.

Fischl knew that the other lingering problem from Covid would either be COPD or Bronchitis. He tests for neither. I was, as I invariably always was, on my own.

By March 7, 2020, I was in such dire straits that I had to go to the hospital. There, they ran the tests that Fischl should have done. And they diagnosed me with an upper respiratory infection coupled with acute bronchitis. And urged me to see Fischl asap (no later than March 10, 2020. Fischl refused to see me and, on March 12 and 13, I attempted to get the one drug that I knew would help me---Gentamicin. Instead, Fischl and his cronies "fired" me and left me to fend for myself. If you ever doubted that the man intentionally caused me harm and sought my demise, there can no longer be any doubt.

I was abandoned with no meds and no medical treatment right smack in the middle of the covid lockdown. I suffered tremendously as I struggled to breath and my blood pressure routinely jumped to 205/110. I had no access to meds and the clinic was refusing to help me.

Until I saw a new doctor on December 17, 2020, at least three symptoms of covid persisted. Coughing, inability to breath, headaches, and periodic fevers. It had been the fevers that drove me to the hospital in the first place.

Dr. Fiorella Saavedra:

95

12/17/2020:   193/105   no pulse listed   297lbs
meds:
1. Amlodipine 2.5mg
2. Irbesartan 300mg
3. Tamsulosin .4mg
4. Received Pneumococcal Polysaccharide shot
5. Spironolactone 25mg
Issues addressed:
1. Essential Hypertension
2. screening for hyperlipidemia
3. BPH with urinary frequency
4. Need for hep C screening test
5. Colon cancer screening
6. Encounter to establish care.

01/06/2021:   144/79   no pulse listed   286lbs
meds:
*prescribed Atorvastatin 20mg (it's a pill they give you for prediabetes to try to prevent dibetes). I could not get it because they had prescribed it through their inhouse pharmacy and I did not have forty dollars to buy it with.

04/27/2021:   136/80   no pulse listed   290lbs
meds:
1. Fio had looked on the chart back in December of 2020, to see what Fischl had been giving me. She now asked me why he had me on Spironolactone and I had no answer. Subsequently, she opted not to give me that and I stopped taking it.
2. Fio had my prescription transferred to Wal-mart. I picked it up for $1.40

As I recall, I quit taking it after two days because it was making me sick. It would become one more thing to hate

Fischl for. While you contemplate that, here's something else for you to ponder, why did Fischl change enlarged prostate to "BHP"? Give up?

Fischl used BHP as an excuse for prescribing the Tamsulosin. In the next chapter, we get to look for more clues as to what Fischl was up to. The most obvious was that, in three years, he never once gave me a PSA test. Why? Because his predecessors had already done so and determined that my prostate was healthy. If he tests, then he has no excuse for prescribing Tamsulosin. Look for yourself.

Prior to all of those water pills, I was peeing, on average, ten to twelve times a day. After the water pills, I was peeing twice that often. It was ridiculous. Urinary frequency? Up yours.

The Tests

The following is a list of tests that my doctors had ordered. In all cases, I list both the name and the date that the test was either ordered or performed. In some cases, as needed, I will list some of the results of those tests. I may even explain the significance of the test and why it was ordered. Let's start with the year 2012 and see if we can establish a pattern of abuse. Keep in mind that the Affordable Health Care Act was signed into law March 23, 2010.

2012:

<u>May 23, 2012</u>: On this date, four labs were ordered up by a Dr. Richard Carl Davies. Do not confuse the word "lab" with "test." A test is a single procedure. A lab can be an order for several tests. The four labs were: CBC with automated differential, Complete Metabolic panel, Prostatic Specific Antigen - Diagnostic, and Urinalysis with microscopic exam.

The PSA test came back with a very respectable, 2.93 -I was 59 years old.

2015:

<u>July 21, 2015</u>: On this date, a Dr. Robert L. Sloan ordered up a lab called Urinalysis with microscopic exam.

I should take a moment out to let you know what is going on because this stuff is at loggerheads with the list of visits. For whatever reason, some visits were deleted from the system. We know this because the tests were not ordered on their own. There had to be a corresponding office visit. Your question should be, as mine is, why?

You should bear in mind that, for every test listed, there was a result. I have copies of most of the results. However, there were tests that were done where no result was forthcoming. Again, we must ask why?

I am not totally sure, but my recollection is that Dr. Davies and Dr. Sloan may have been employed at an Urgent Care clinic. I may be wrong. On the other hand, I am positive that Dr. Brett Hayes (11-10-2015 to 11-14-2016) and Dr. Mark Fischl (02-16-2017 to 01-31-2020) were, at all material times herein, employed at the Salem Clinic. And so we now look at the tests ordered by each of those two doctors and the dates thereof.

<u>November 10, 2015</u>:
1. Syphilis
2. Lipid Profile (screen)
3. Glycohemoglobin (A1C)
4. Complete Metabolic Panel
5. HIV-1 & HIV-2 Antibody
6. Hepatitis Panel Chronic (Reflexive)

* Syphilis? HIV? I was in my 60s and hadn't had sex in ten years. These tests were unnecessary. But, as I said, they make the clinic, and the doctor, money.

December 4, 2015:
1. Prostatic Specific Antigen (screen). Result: 3.89 (great). I was 62.

2016:

November 14, 2016:
1. Fecal Occult Blood - CCO

2017:

February 16, 2017:
1. Magnesium - serum
2. Basic Metabolic Panel
3. CBC with automated differential

March 7, 2017:
1. Basic Metabolic Panel

May 19, 2017:
1. Basic Metabolic Panel

May 23, 2017:
1. XR Post Void Residual

August 21, 2017:
1. Magnesium - serum
2. Basic Metabolic Panel

November 28, 2017:
1. Basic Metabolic Panel
2. Lipid Profile (screen)

December 22, 2017:
1. Fecal Occult Blood (FIT) Diagnostic

2018:

April 2, 2018:
1. Aldosterone/Renin Ratio
2. Basic Metabolic Panel

July 3, 2018:
1. Basic Metabolic Panel

2019:

March 21, 2019:
1. Basic Metabolic Panel

July 16, 2019:
1. Renal Function Panel
2. Thoracic/Lumbar Spine X-ray

2020:

January 31, 2020:
1. Influenza A + B Antigen (Rapid)

March 7, 2020:
These tests were done at Salem Hospital and ordered by Dr. Lazeni Koulibali. Unlike Fischl, instead of guessing what he thought I had and then testing for it, Dr. Koulibali ordered a broad spectrum of tests and went looking for my ailment.
1. Complete Metabolic Panel
2. CBC with automated differential

3. Chest x-ray.

Although I had a diagnosis for Bronchitis and upper respiratory infection, I received no medical treatment for that diagnosis. Fischl had fired me for demanding that he treat me with something. We were on lockdown and I was unable to find a new doctor until December 17, 2020. On this date, my new doctor, Fiorella Saavedra, ordered the following labs:

December 17, 2020:

1. Complete Metabolic Panel with GFR
2. CBC with auto differential
3. Hemoglobin A1C
4. Lipid Panel
5. Prostatic Specific Antigen (PSA) test
6. HVC AB, Reflex RT-PCR
7. Interpretation

* Fischl never did order a PSA test and had no way of knowing if my prostate was abnormal or not. Here, under the care of Fio, my PSA was 5.6. It was flagged as high. But there were things that had skewed the test. Sex within two days, the Tamsulosin, dehydration, bacterial infection, and parasites. Additionally, for a 67 year old man, 5.6 was reasonable.

2021:

April 27, 2021:
1. Hemoglobin A1C
2. PSA

* Here my PSA had dropped back down to 4.6. There was,

103

literally, nothing to be concerned with. And yet, for three years, Fischl had treated me for it. Again, without ever testing.

May 6, 2021:
1. Fecal Occult Blood (FIT)

July 29, 2021:
1. Complete Metabolic Panel (14) with GFR
2. CBC with auto differential
3. H. Pylori AG, stool
4. Ova and Parasite examination
5. Giardia antigen
6. Culture, stool

August 24, 2021:
   After referral to a Urologist, I saw John M. Mhoon and he ordered the usual test.
1. PSA was 8.8. When Mhoon wanted to book me into the hospital and operate, I accused him of having skewed the test results. He got angry and wrote me a slip and told me to retake the test when I thought it was okay. So I waited until after I finished the antibiotics for the bacterial infection, abstained from sex, and drank lots of water. I retook the test on or about September 2, 2021.

September 2, 2021:
1. PSA: 4.34 (less than half of what the skewed test had been). It is worth noting that this result would be respectable for a man in his forties. I promptly fired Mhoon.

October 12, 2021:

104

The tests Fiorella ordered on July 29 had revealed that I was suffering from h. pylori (a bacterial infection) and blastocysts (parasites). After many delays, I finally received the meds, finished treatment and needed tested to see if the meds had worked. Subsequently:
1. H. Pylori AG, stool
2. Ova and parasite examination

The tests revealed that the pylori was gone but not the parasites. I was given more drugs. Today is November 23, 2021, as I write this part of the book. I believe the parasites are gone this time as my appetite has returned and my body is repairing itself. I will be getting tested soon.

In the next chapter, I am going to explain what I was suffering from (since 2016) and what the doctors, particularly Mr. Mark Fischl, did to me...not to cure me but, rather, to make me ill.

For those of you curious about the tests and what they were supposed to be for, I now list them, alphabetically (instead of chronologically), for your perusal.

Labs and Tests Explanations

Aldosterone:
Aldosterone is the main mineralocorticoid steroid hormone produced by the zona glomerulosa of the adrenal cortex in the adrenal gland. It is essential for sodium conservation in the kidney, salivary glands, sweat glands, and colon.

In hyperaldosteronism, overproduction of aldosterone leads to fluid retention and increased blood pressure, weakness, and, rarely, periods of paralysis. Hyperaldosteronism can be caused by a tumor in the adrenal gland or may be a response to some diseases.

In other words, the Aldosterone test was to try to pinpoint the exact cause, or causes, of my high blood pressure.

Aldosterone/Renin Ratio:

Aldosterone-to-renin ratio (ARR) is the mass concentration of aldosterone divided by the plasma renin activity or by serum renin concentration in blood. The aldosterone/renin ratio is recommended as screening tool for primary hyperaldosteronism.

Again, this was a test to try to ascertain why my bp was high. It would become pivotal in proving that Fischl was out to cause me bodily harm. Why? Because I had normal Aldosterone and five times the normal rate for renin. Fischl disregarded this and treated me for high Aldosterone and high renin. It's in black and white. Let's see him deny it.

Basic Metabolic Panel:

A basic metabolic panel is a blood test consisting of a set of seven or eight biochemical tests and is one of the most common lab tests ordered by health care providers.

A comprehensive (I referred to this as "complete") metabolic panel (CMP) is a test that measures 14 different substances in your blood. It provides important information about your body's chemical balance and metabolism. Metabolism is the process of how the body uses food and energy. A CMP includes tests for the following:

Glucose, a type of sugar and your body's main source of energy.
Calcium, one of the body's most important minerals. Calcium is essential for proper functioning of your nerves, muscles, and heart.
Sodium, potassium, carbon dioxide, and chloride. These are

electrolytes, electrically charged minerals that help control the amount of fluids and the balance of acids and bases in your body.

Albumin, a protein made in the liver.

Total protein, which measures the total amount of protein in the blood.

ALP (alkaline phosphatase), ALT (alanine transaminase), and AST (aspartate aminotransferase). These are different enzymes made by the liver.

Bilirubin, a waste product made by the liver.

BUN (blood urea nitrogen) and creatinine, waste products removed from your blood by your kidneys.

Abnormal levels of any of these substances or combination of them can be a sign of a serious health problem.

CBC with automated differential:

A CBC with differential is used to help diagnose and monitor many different conditions, including anemia and infection. Also called blood cell count with differential.

Chest X-ray:

self-explanatory

Complete Metabolic Panel:

Already explained above.

Complete Metabolic Panel with GFR:

GFR stands for glomerular filtration rate. GFR is a measure of how well your kidneys filter blood.

Culture, Stool:

A stool culture is a test on a stool sample to find germs (such as bacteria or a fungus) that can cause an infection. A sample of stool is added to a substance that promotes the growth of germs. If no germs grow, the culture is negative. If germs that can cause infection grow, the culture is positive.

Fecal Occult Blood - CCO:

The fecal occult blood test (FOBT) is a lab test used to check stool samples for hidden (occult) blood. Occult blood in the stool may indicate colon cancer or polyps in the colon or rectum — though not all cancers or polyps bleed.

GFR:

GFR stands for glomerular filtration rate. GFR is a measure of how well your kidneys filter blood.

Giardia Antigen:

The Giardia lamblia parasite is one of the chief causes of diarrhea in the United States. It lives in the gastrointestinal (GI) system and passes from the body in stool (feces).

In a Giardia antigen test, a stool sample is checked for the presence of Giardia.

Glycohemoglobin (A1C):

The hemoglobin A1c test tells you your average level of blood sugar over the past 2 to 3 months. It's also called HbA1c, glycated hemoglobin

H. Pylori AG, Stool:

The most common stool test to detect H. pylori is called a stool antigen test that looks for foreign proteins (antigens) associated with H. pylori infection in your stool. Antibiotics, acid-suppressing drugs known as proton pump inhibitors (PPIs) and bismuth subsalicylate (Pepto-Bismol) can interfere with the accuracy of these tests.

Hemoglobin A1C:
    See glycohemoglobin.

Hepatitis Panel Chronic (reflexive):
    A hepatitis panel is a blood test that checks to see if you have a hepatitis infection caused by one of these viruses. The viruses are spread in different ways and cause different symptoms: Hepatitis A is most often spread by contact with contaminated feces (stool) or by eating tainted food.
    If the term "w/reflex" is listed in your test results, this means that the blood test was repeated to confirm a positive result on your first hepatitis blood test. A positive result may mean that you have hepatitis antibodies from a recent infection.

HIV-1 & HIV-2 Antibody:
    The HIV antibody test advised by the CDC is the HIV-1/2 antigen/antibody combination immunoassay test. If you test positive for HIV, the CDC advises the following follow-up tests: HIV-1/HIV-2 antibody differentiation immunoassay. This test is to confirm HIV and find out if you have HIV-1 or HIV-2.

HVC AB, Reflex RT-PCR:
    Hepatitis C Antibody with Reflex to HCV RNA,PCR w/Reflex to Genotype, LiPA - Hepatitis C Virus (HCV) is the major cause of hepatitis. Making positive HCV Ab tests reflex to confirmatory molecular testing is necessary to confirm active HCV infection.

Influenza A + B Antigen (rapid):
    Test for the two major flu bugs

Interpretation:
General q & a with doctor as to test results and/or general health of patient.

Lipid Profile (screen):
Diagnostic evaluation of diseases associated with altered lipid metabolism, such as: nephrotic syndrome, pancreatitis, hepatic disease, and hypo and hyperthyroidism. Secondary dyslipidemia, including diabetes mellitus, disorders of gastrointestinal absorption, chronic renal failure.

Fats and lipids are an essential component of the homeostatic function of the human body. Lipids contribute to some of the body's most vital processes. Lipids are fatty, waxy, or oily compounds that are soluble in organic solvents and insoluble in polar solvents such as water.

Magnesium - Serum:
A magnesium blood test is used to check the level of magnesium in your blood. Levels that are too low are known as hypomagnesemia or magnesium

Ova and Parasite Examination:
An ova and parasite test looks for parasites and their eggs (ova) in a sample of your stool. A parasite is a tiny plant or animal that gets nutrients by living off another creature. Parasites can live in your digestive system and cause illness. These are known as intestinal parasites.

Prostatic Specific Antigen:
The PSA test is a blood test to help detect prostate cancer. But it's not perfect and will not find all prostate cancers. The test, which can be done at a GP surgery, measures the level of prostate-specific antigen (PSA) in your blood. PSA is a

protein made only by the prostate gland.

Renal Function Panel:
A renal panel is a group of tests that may be performed together to evaluate kidney (renal) function. The tests measure levels of various substances:

Panel includes albumin, calcium, carbon dioxide, creatinine, chloride, glucose, phosphorous, potassium, sodium, and BUN and a calculated anion gap value.

Syphillis:
self-explanatory

Thoracic/Lumbar Spine X-ray:
self-explanatory

Urinalysis with Microscopic Exam:
This test looks at a sample of your urine under a microscope. It can see cells from your urinary tract, blood cells, crystals, bacteria, parasites, and cells from tumors. This test is often used to confirm the findings of other tests or add information to a diagnosis.

XR Post Void Residual:
The post-void residual (PVR) urine test measures the amount of urine left in the bladder after urination. The test is used to help evaluate: Incontinence (accidental release of urine) in women and men.

111

Medical Malpractice & Negligence

I seriously considered calling this chapter Fischl's Thistles or some equally catchy phrase. While many of the things in this chapter apply to most all doctors, they primarily apply to Mark Fischl as he purposely used drugs to facilitate various ailments and afflictions so that he could play hero---the very definition of Munchausen's.

Fischl's predecessor, Dr. Brett Hayes, was a much younger man and dedicated to his craft and his patients. On or about November 18 of 2016, Dr. Hayes realized that I was suffering from dehydration (in large part because I was experiencing high blood pressure, weight loss, and an elevated pulse) and sought to get a handle on that by stopping two of the water pills most responsible for that condition. He stopped the hydrochlorothiazide and the Tamsulosin (Flomax).

On that day, Dr. Hayes had noted that he was seeing me for BPH. It was the last time that he would even consider it, and would downgrade the prognosis to enlarged Prostate. The difference? An enlarged prostate is a normal fact of life for elderly men. If it exists without causing problems, it is just enlarged and nothing else. However, if it causes any of the following symptoms, it gets raised to BPH (Benign Prostatic Hyperplasia).

1. Frequent or urgent need to urinate.
2. Increased frequency of urination at night (nocturia)
3. Difficulty starting urination.
4. Weak urine stream or a stream that stops and starts.
5. Dribbling at the end of urination.
6. Inability to completely empty the bladder.

The following are some of the symptoms for dehydration.

1. feeling thirsty.
2. dark yellow and strong-smelling pee.
3. feeling dizzy or lightheaded.
4. feeling tired.
5. a dry mouth, lips and eyes.
6. peeing little, and fewer than 4 times a day.

As you can plainly see, by prescribing water pills all the time, the doctors could not rely on the last symptom on that list because water pills make you pee all the time. This is especially true of Flomax. That is why Dr. Hayes stopped the drug.

What is a diuretic? Diuretics, also known as water pills, are medicines that help you move extra fluid and salt out of your body. They make you pee more frequently, which is why you should take them in the morning if you can.

These drugs treat high blood pressure and heart failure. They do it by helping your kidneys produce more urine. The more you pee, the more excess salt and water you flush out of your body. Without the extra fluid, it's easier for your heart to pump. While they may help your body get rid of extra fluid, they can sometimes dehydrate you, which can be bad for your kidneys.

Ok, but how could Hayes have known that? The most

obvious signs of dehydration were the high blood pressure, that sometimes didn't seem to be responding well to drugs, and the second, and most obvious, was merely the high pulse rate.

In the world of medicine, there are several things that can cause an elevated pulse. Anxiety, fear, exercise, dehydration, heart trouble, and a bacterial infection. For an old man with high blood pressure, as a doctor, I would have been looking at the heart. But Fischl never does. Why? Because he already knew I was suffering from dehydration.

Obviously, Fischl is going to vehemently deny any such allegations. Talk, as they say, is cheap. They also say that actions speak louder than words. That is why I pointed out that Fischl was never concerned with my heart...and this was in total disregard of what my symptoms were telling him. I.E. High blood pressure, shortness of breath, etc.

Sometimes inaction becomes action. By not taking the appropriate steps (tests), Fischl could not rule out my heart. However, due to the influence of Munchausen's, the man thought himself to be a demigod or messiah. All he had to do was look into his crystal ball and see if my heart was okay. Amazing.

The first time I ever met Fischl was February of 2017. On that date, in that place, my blood pressure was a very respectable 113/81. My pulse, on the other hand, was elevated at 85 beats per minute. We already know what Fischl didn't do, but what, exactly, did our hero do?

On or about February 16, 2017, Mark R. Fischl knows that his predecessor, Dr Hayes, had me on two water pills. I was taking Chlorthalidone 100mg and Spironolactone 25mg. Water pills are notorious for making you pee a lot. Let's look at Fischl's diagnosis.

On that date, Fischl noted the following:

1. Essential (primary) hypertension
2. Urinary frequency
3. Enlarged prostate without luts (lower urinary tract symptoms)
4. Hypokalemia

Fischl knows that the hypokalemia was a direct consequence of peeing all the time. It prevented my body from absorbing the necessary amount of potassium from the foods I ingested. What I find particularly interesting is right after he lists urinary frequency, he writes that I had an enlarged prostate without luts. Why is that so interesting? Urinary frequency is one of the symptoms (luts) that he was claiming I did not have.

Obviously, we want to know what Fischl was doing about the water pills and the resultant urinary frequency. He should be commended for cutting the Chlorthalidone in half. Then he should be strung up for what he does next. Huh? Fischl promptly prescribed the worst water pill ever invented.

There I was, near-perfect blood pressure, suffering from dehydration, my potassium level was dropping from urinary frequency, and Fischl prescribes a third water pill? What the hell?

Tamsulosin is the drug from hell. It is a massive water pill that works by relaxing the muscles in both your prostate and your bladder. The theory held by most doctors is that by relaxing those muscles, it allows you to expel most of the liquid in your bladder and that is suppose to make you pee less often. Unfortunately, just the opposite happens. And I'm going to tell you why.

It is a medical fact that when you do not use muscles, they tend to atrophy. What that means is they get lazy and can't do their job. In english? It means that the prostate muscle relaxes and cannot contain the prostate. The prostate gets bigger. But the more serious problem is that the bladder muscles can't hold very much water with relaxed muscles.

All of that is bad enough, in and of itself, but there is one more problem that needs addressed. As those muscles relax, they get more sensitive. In the real world, that translates to frequent urination because the bladder senses the slightest increase in water and feels compelled to expel it. This is especially noticeable when you lay down (hence "nocturia").

Because the muscles are relaxed, they atrophy and lose their ability to hold back urine. At this point in the patient's life, he/she experiences incontinence. It is something almost any medical student knows but, thanks to the almighty dollar, doctors like to ignore while they peddle more and more drugs. Profitability.

When Fischl sees me again, three months later, he notes the following problems:
1. Urinary frequency-primary
2. Essential (primary) hypertension.

"Primary" is a medical term denoting an unknown cause. Excuse me! WTF! Three water pills and the clown cannot figure out why I was peeing so much? Surely you jest.

The good news was that my pulse had dropped from 85 beats per minute to 77bpm. The bad news, as expected, was that my blood pressure had jumped up to 150/77. Now I am no doctor, but I have studied enough medicine to predict that those stats would have done precisely what they did. How?

When a person is dehydrated, they can experience either high blood pressure or an elevated pulse. At other times, a person may be experiencing both. It is also possible that, I was hydrated on that day and my pulse dropped. The increase blood pressure could have been residual or caused by

117

something else (such as pain).

Before we resume with what Fischl was, or wasn't doing, I want to take a side excursion so as to explain the role of the kidneys, bladder, and their relationship to the enlarged prostate. This is important because, so far, you think everything that was going on was somewhat understandable. But that was not the truth. Let's look at why.

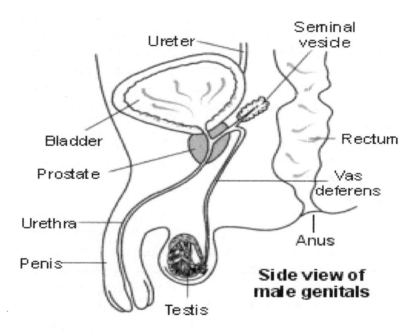

In the above diagram, at the top, you see a tube called the Ureter. The ureter is a tube that carries urine from the kidney to the urinary bladder. There are two ureters, one attached to each kidney. The upper half of the ureter is located in the abdomen and the lower half is located in the pelvic area.

A ureteral obstruction is a blockage in one or both of the

118

tubes (ureters) that carry urine from your kidneys to your bladder. Ureteral obstruction can be curable. However, if it's not treated, symptoms can quickly move from mild — pain, fever and infection — to severe — loss of kidney function, sepsis and death.

Symptoms of a blocked ureter or urinary tract obstruction include:

1. Pain in your abdomen, lower back or sides below your ribs (flank pain).
2. Fever, nausea or vomiting.
3. Difficulty urinating or emptying your bladder.
4. Frequent urination.
5. Recurring urinary tract infections (UTI).
6. Urine that is bloody or cloudy.

Your kidneys make urine by filtering wastes and extra water from your blood. The urine travels from the kidneys to the bladder in two thin tubes called ureters.

The ureters are about 8 to 10 inches long. Muscles in the ureter walls tighten and relax to force urine down and away from the kidneys. Small amounts of urine flow from the ureters into the bladder about every 10 to 15 seconds.

Sometimes the ureters can become blocked or injured. This can block the flow of urine to the bladder. If urine stands still or backs up the ureter, you may get urinary tract infections.

Doctors diagnose problems with the ureters using different tests. These include urine tests, x-rays, and examination of the ureter with a scope called a cystoscope. Treatment depends on the cause of the problem. It may include medicines and, in severe cases, surgery.

On May 19, 2017, Fischl ordered a test called XR Post Void Residual. The test was done on May 23, 2017. To date, late 2021, I have been unable to obtain the results. The online site that is supposed to reveal this to me, simply states no component available. I click on images and none show up.

The Void test was supposed to measure how much urine remained in my bladder once I voided, or expelled, urine. If a patient has high post-void residual volume of urine left in the bladder, it could indicate a urinary tract infection, a renal deficiency or benign prostatic hyperplasia(BPH).

We can look at what Fischl did or didn't do when I saw him three months later, on August 21, 2017. I see no clue as to what was, or wasn't, revealed in the Void test. Virtually everything I was diagnosed with was something revealed by the other test Fischl had ordered on May 19. Basic Metabolic Panel. The diagnosis?

1. Hypokalemia
2. Essential (primary) hypertension
3. Urinary frequency
4. Elevated Lipids
5. Need for hepatitis screening.

I was starting to see a pattern. Fischl would adjust my meds so as to create a problem and then conduct more tests or prescribe more pills to make more money. What? Have you already forgotten that doctors are first, and foremost, businessmen. They threw up a shingle, opened an office, hired staff, and all that such a business entails. To pay for that, they must do something.

Just as an example, because we do not know exact fees, let's analyze a typical visit. Now, if you simply went to a doctor and he prescribed neither a test nor a drug, the base charge might be a hundred dollars. If he prescribes either a test or a drug, he can tack on another hundred. Simultaneously, his buddy at the laboratory gets to charge you for that visit. Win-win for everybody...except the patient.

But doesn't the insurance company lose, too? That depends on a lot of factors. With the advent of mandatory health insurance for everybody, the government actually foots the bill or, at the very least, subsidizes some portion of the expense. So the insurance companies are getting rich, too. If they were not getting rich, they would not be in business, now would they?

So my doctor(s) put me on water pills that cause things like urinary frequency. That, in turn, causes things like low potassium (hypokalemia) and elevated lipids. These, in turn, justify my doctors repeatedly testing for hepatitis. More money.

High lipid levels may also be caused by medical conditions such as diabetes, hypothyroidism, alcoholism, kidney disease, liver disease and stress. In some people, certain medicines, such as birth control pills, steroids and blood pressure medicines, can cause high lipid levels. Who would have thunk it?

And what is hepatitis? Hepatitis means inflammation of the liver. The liver is a vital organ that processes nutrients, filters the blood, and fights infections. Heavy alcohol use, toxins, some medications, and certain medical conditions can cause hepatitis. However, hepatitis is often caused by a virus.

The primary functions of the liver are:
1. Bile production and excretion.
2. Excretion of bilirubin, cholesterol, hormones, and drugs.
3. Metabolism of fats, proteins, and carbohydrates.
4. Enzyme activation.
5. Storage of glycogen, vitamins, and minerals.
6. Synthesis of plasma proteins, such as albumin, and clotting factors.

So far, under the overabundance of pills prescribed by

121

Fischl, we have him looking for excuses to treat just about every organ in my body. He is treating the prostate, the kidneys, the heart, and trying to add bladder and liver to the laundry list. The more pills, the longer the list becomes. Not only does Fischl get to play hero, he gets lots of money doing so. What a racket.

Prior to the water pills, there was no hypokalemia. Prior to the water pills, there was no low potassium. Prior to Fischl, there was no elevated lipids. Instead of my health improving, it was deteriorating due to medical intervention. This malpractice was unnecessary and unjustified. Let's look at the test results obtained by Fischl the very first time I saw him (February 16, 2017).

Fischl had ordered a Basic Metabolic Panel, a CBC with automated differential, and a magnesium test. The results of the Basic metabolic panel showed that my potassium level had dipped slightly, my carbon dioxide levels were high, and my calcium level was a tad high. The result of the CBC showed that my red blood cell count was high, my hematocrit level was high, MPV pegged the top of "normal," and monocytes were high. Magnesium was a touch above normal.

What does all of that mean in english? MPV stands for mean platelet volume. Platelets are small blood cells that are essential for blood clotting, the process that helps you stop bleeding after an injury. An MPV blood test measures the average size of your platelets. The test can help diagnose bleeding disorders and diseases of the bone marrow.

Of interest to us at this stage of the game is the high hematocrit level. A higher than normal hematocrit can indicate: Dehydration. It can also be a disorder, such as polycythemia vera, that causes your body to produce too many red blood cells. Lung or heart disease. The question arises, why didn't Fischl address the dehydration issue that was screaming at him? And the biggest question of them all is why, when my blood pressure was so ideal, 113/81, did Fischl take such drastic steps to mess it all up?

In case you missed it, dehydration causes both the high hematocrit level and the high red blood cell count that were measured in the laboratory. Was Fischl too busy looking into his crystal ball?

Apparently his crystal ball was not fine tuned to deal with high carbon dioxide levels, either. Hypercapnia, or hypercarbia, is a condition that arises from having too much carbon dioxide in the blood. It is often caused by hypoventilation or disordered breathing where not enough oxygen enters the lungs and not enough carbon dioxide is emitted. There are other causes of hypercapnia, as well, including some lung diseases.

Hypercapnia symptoms can range from mild to severe. There are many potential causes of hypercapnia. The following are considered to be mild symptoms of hypercapnia:

1. dizziness
2. drowsiness
3. excessive fatigue
4. headaches
5. feeling disoriented
6. flushing of the skin
7. shortness of breath

These symptoms of hypercapnia may arise from shorter periods of shallow or slow breathing, such as during deep sleep. They may not always be a cause for concern, as the body is often able to correct the symptoms and balance carbon dioxide levels in the bloodstream without intervention.

However, if the above symptoms persist for several days, it is advisable to see a doctor.

The symptoms of severe hypercapnia require immediate medical attention, as they can cause long-term complications. Some cases may be fatal.

Severe hypercapnia symptoms include:

1. confusion
2. coma
3. depression or paranoia
4. hyperventilation or excessive breathing
5. irregular heartbeat or arrhythmia
6. loss of consciousness
7. muscle twitching
8. panic attacks
9. seizures

There are many causes of hypercapnia including the following:

Chronic obstructive pulmonary disease or COPD:

COPD is an umbrella term for several conditions that affect the breathing. Common forms of COPD include chronic bronchitis and emphysema. Chronic bronchitis leads to inflammation and mucus in the airways, while emphysema involves damage to the air sacs or alveoli in the lungs. Both conditions can cause increased levels of carbon dioxide in the bloodstream.

The main cause of COPD is long-term exposure to lung irritants. According to the National Heart, Lung, and Blood InstituteTrusted Source, cigarette smoke is the most common lung irritant that causes COPD in the United States. Air pollution and exposure to chemicals or dust may also cause COPD.

Although not everyone with COPD will develop hypercapnia, a person's risk increases as their COPD progresses.

Sleep apnea:

The National Sleep Foundation reports that between 5 and 20 percent of adults have sleep apnea. This common condition is characterized by shallow breathing, or pauses in breathing, during sleep. It can interfere with the level of oxygen in the bloodstream and throw off the body's balance of carbon dioxide and oxygen.

Sleep apnea symptoms include:

1. daytime sleepiness
2. headaches upon waking
3. difficulty concentrating
4. snoring

Genetics:

Rarely, a genetic condition where the liver fails to produce enough alpha-1-antitrypsin (AAT) can cause hypercapnia. Alpha-1-antitrypsin is a protein that is necessary for lung health, so AAT deficiency is a risk factor for COPD development.

Nerve disorders and muscular problems:

In some people, the nerves and muscles necessary for proper lung function may not work correctly. For example, muscular dystrophy can cause the muscles to weaken, eventually leading to breathing problems.

Other disorders of the nervous or muscular systems that can contribute to hypercapnia include:

1. Amyotrophic lateral sclerosis (ALS), a progressive disease that affects nerve cells in the brain and spinal cord.
2. Encephalitis or when a person has inflammation of the brain.
3. Guillain-Barré syndrome that can be caused by an abnormal immune response.
4. Myasthenia gravis, a chronic disease that can weaken the skeletal muscles responsible for breathing.

Other causes of high blood levels of carbon dioxide include:

1. Activities that impact breathing, including diving or ventilator use.
2. Brainstem stroke, which can affect breathing.
3. Hypothermia, a medical emergency caused by rapid heat loss from the body.
4. Obesity hypoventilation syndromes when overweight people cannot breathe deeply or quickly enough.
5. An overdose of certain drugs, such as opioids or benzodiazepines.

During the COVID-19 pandemic, some people are concerned that wearing a face mask could lead to hypercapnia. However, there is very little evidence to suggest that face masks can cause hypercapnia.

Author's note:
I believe that there is little evidence to support that a mask increases carbon dioxide levels. This may be true or it may be because nobody has tested the hypothesis. Either way, masks do hinder a person's ability to breath and thus reduce the amount of oxygen they inhale. This, in turn, will affect the ratio of carbon dioxide to oxygen in the body...and that isn't good.

Face masks are not airtight, and they are made out of materials that allow airflow. This allows carbon dioxide to circulate rather than build up. Even medical grade N95 fitted masks allow carbon dioxide flow, which makes it unlikely that any significant amount of the gas will build up.

Thinner surgical and cloth masks are more porous and loose fitting, which allows for even more air exchange.

The Centers for Disease Control and Protection (CDC)Trusted Source recommend that a person only wears a mask when going out in public or when around people who do not live in their household to help prevent the spread of COVID-19. Excess carbon dioxide does not build up during these short windows of time (the inference being that they do over prolonged periods).

Anyone who has difficulty breathing is not required to wear a face mask. (this last comment was from the CDC themselves. So why haven't we heard about it on television, on the internet, or anywhere? Masks are killing people.)

For the next two years, Fischl would play around with my meds. Though there was ample evidence proving that I was dehydrated and suffering from a bacterial infection, Fischl remained oblivious to my plight. He had it in his brain that I was old, I was fat, and, at least in his mind, lazy. Even so, he ignored my heart; choosing only to prescribe blood pressure medication.

Fischl's obsession and lack of vision was causing my health to deteriorate on multiple levels. He notes that I suffered from chronic back pain (not associated with the sciatic nerve). And, eventually, orders x-rays (on July 16, 2019). While they showed that I had osteophytes on each of my vertebra, that did not adequately explain what was going on. More tests were in order but none came. Apparently Fischl not a very good businessman either.

When I saw Fischl on or about October 17, 2019, I informed him that my back pain was decreasing because I was drinking cranberry juice (for a UTI that he rarely, if ever, tested for). His response had been to tell me "placebo effect." Just as he had repeatedly disregarded the symptoms of dehydration, he was now disregarding the symptoms of a bacterial infection; not just the symptoms, but also the cure.

That I was responding to the cranberry juice clearly establish the presence of some kind of bacterial infection. Wheras it was not, necessarily, the result of a Urinary Tract Infection, it existed nonetheless. No tests; only insults. Placebo effect.

From that day forward, my health would spiral rapidly downhill. It was not necessary. It should not have happened. But I had a doctor that was too busy patting himself on the back. In itself, not so bad. But Fischl refused to listen to me. My life was about to get worse; much worse.

Education verses Experience

Earlier, I explained that there are two types of people in this world. One type, exemplified by Mark Fischl, consists of memorizing textbooks and whatnot. These kinds of people lack the ability to think and do not readily process information. In Fischl's case, he knew that putting me on water pills would dehydrate me even further than I was and cause damages to my kidneys, liver, and all the rest. We know this because he was continually looking for it.

The second kind of people are the processor types. These are the thinkers who invent things to benefit mankind. I belong to this classification. I process information on complex levels.

At the time that I was seeing Fischl, I was trusting him. It wasn't until he told me "placebo effect" that I started to realize that he was not a very nice man...and an even worse doctor. Oh, there had been other signs; things to which he made lame excuses. Pitiful.

I once asked him for twelve vicodan for my back pain. Why twelve? I was working in a flea market once a month. On those days, I would experience excruciating back pain from the hard concrete floor. You people with back problems know exactly what I'm talking about. Anyway, whenever it was time to pack my stuff up and take it to my car, I would be in so much pain that I could not do it. On those days, I would have to pay someone to do it for me. It was money that I couldn't afford to spend and twelve pills, in theory, would solve that dilemma.

Instead of prescribing the pills, Fischl notes that I was a drug seeker. The term is a negative one used to say a person is a drug addict. Excuse me, asshole, but how many goddamned drug addicts do you know who only ask for twelve frigging pills a year? Drug seeker? Placebo effect? F@#k you Fischl.

Another time I asked Fischl to fill out a form so I could get a handicapped parking permit from the Department of Motor Vehicles. At the time, I could barely walk and I had to use a shopping cart just to get to the door of the supermarket. Fischl turned a deaf ear to my plight and insisted that the law stated that he could not issue me such a form unless I had to have a cane or a walker. Asshole.

I had lower back pain. His premise was that I should have been using a cane or a walker. Excuse me dumbass, people who claim to have lower back pain and use walkers or canes are, in my experience, fakers. When I broke my back in an automobile accident, I tried walking with those things. I even tried crutches. Nope, no good. The problem? When you use those things, because your lower back is a fulcrum, it increases pressure on your lower back and that increases pain exponentially. Kiss my ass.

Another excuse used by Fischl was that he could not issue one unless I was not able to walk 200 feet without aid of some kind. Bingo, we have a winner. I used a shopping cart. However, because I had not used one of them to get into his office, he denied me. Let me enlighten you and him. All of those sonsofbitches claiming bad backs could walk 200 feet without canes or walkers. Every single lousy one of them. You see, if you can walk that far with a cane or walker, you can walk that far without one. Scientific fact and a medical certainty.

My opinion of Fischl was that he was a womanizer. If one of those poor dears hobbled in, he couldn't help them fast enough. But let a man all but crawl in there and he denies all treatment and all semblance of human decency.

To say that my first two years with Fischl was a hellish experience would be a severe understatement of facts. Even so, they pale in comparison to what he would ultimately do to me. I never imagined that a medical professional could be so heartless. How wrong I was.

I had gotten covid 19 in December of 2019. It peaked on January 6, 2020. When I say peaked, I am referencing the fact that I lost all sense of taste and smell. Absent any other information, I cannot say that January 6, 2020 was at the end of the covid, or nearer to the beginning. Nor can I say, with any certainty, that covid lasted two weeks, three weeks, or is, in fact, ongoing.

According to Fischl's crystal ball, covid lasts 10 to 14 days. I'm going to call bullshit on that one as there have been, and are, people in the hospital who routinely have it for a month or more. Be that as it may, I saw Fischl on January 31, 2020.

"The things I'm experiencing are unlike anything I've ever had," I said resolutely.

As always, I might as well have been talking to the wall. Fischl disregarded everything I said and orders tests for influenza A and influenza B. Goddamn it, I know what the flu feels like. Hello? Is anybody home?

As expected, I tested negative for the flu bug. Next? There was no next. With Fischl, there never was a next. He would look into his crystal ball, determine what I was suffering from, and then test for that something. It was a crap shoot;

fifty-fifty. And I was losing.

With no further tests, and unable to breath, I struggled until my relatives threatened to tie me up and haul me into the hospital. On March 7, 2020, I capitulated and went to Salem Hospital. On that Saturday, I was fortunate enough to get a real doctor; one that was not afraid to admit that he did not know what was wrong. And he ordered up a battery of tests.

March 7, 2020, had been a Saturday (night). It only took an hour or so for the attending physician to figure out that I was suffering from an upper respiratory infection and acute bronchitis. Upon release from the hospital, I was admonished to see Fischl asap; no later than three days from then.

On Monday morning, March 9, 2020, I went to Salem Clinic and attempted to see Fischl. I told the receptionist what was going on and she went back to talk to Fischl in person. About fifteen minutes later, she returned and informed me that Fischl could not see me that day. She assured me that they would contact me with a date and time.

Three more days passed. I was really struggling to breath. As per his usual disassociative self, Fischl continued to decline to see me. Finally, in desperation, I sent him a message through the online program, Mychart, asking him for Gentamicin. Specifically, I wanted it in a liquid form so I could aerate it. At the time, I did not know that Gentamicin also came in a nebulizer. Fischl knew, but continued to disregard my serious situation and left me to die.

Still don't think Fischl was trying to kill me? Let me remove all doubts. Instead of prescribing something to help me breath and/or cure my respiratory ailments, Fischl goes to his bosses at Salem Clinic and these criminals conspired to deny me all medical attention by sending me a certified letter informing me that Fischl was no longer going to see me as a patient and neither would Salem Clinic, et al (fancy lawyer

132

words for and all).

The letter was signed and dated March 17, 2020, and I think I received it a few weeks later. Shortly after that, thanks to the covid scare, everything went on lockdown. In essence, I had no doctor and, hence, no medical treatment. Nor could I get a new doctor or treatment because doctors were not seeing their old patients...let alone new ones. That was, potentially, a death sentence.

Ironically, in their letter, they stated that Fischl was no longer going to see me because of the "lack of a patient/doctor relationship. That was most certainly true, but they fired the wrong guy.

Here's the deal. A doctor can only be as good as his patient. Why? Because I have lived with me all of my life. I know every nuance of my medical record. A doctor does not have the time nor desire to look up every little detail regarding my history. In that sense, I am more knowledgeable than the doctor.

Am I a doctor? No, that's why I seek out physicians to assist me. I have a genius I.Q. and can make educated guesses as to what I think may be wrong, but the doctor has both the education and the experience to address any supposition. Or, at least, that is the way it is supposed to work. Unfortunately, Fischl suffered a severe disconnect due to his inflated ego in which he considered/considers his patients to be beneath him.

In his online response to my attempts to get treated, he lectures me about what he thinks he knows about covid 19. How nice that he read literature about it, but, at the time, there really wasn't much known about it. And so anything he assumed was more or less invalid. At the very least, anything he read was going to amount to squat next to my actual experiences with that affliction.

Fischl erroneously thinks that Covid just comes and goes.

And yet I, like million of others, suffered from symptoms known as "long covid." No sir. My covid did not merely come and go.

But let's forget that for the time being and look at the main problem. Whether covid or not, I was suffering from an upper respiratory infection and acute bronchitis. Fischl has the hospital records in front of his face. Moreover, I alluded to those records. There was no disconnect on my part. I was forthcoming and trying to get his attention. Yes, Virginia, there was a lack of doctor/patient relationship. It was because there was no doctor.

Absent any help, and knowing full well that I could not get any help, I began asking around. First, I acquired a partial dose of amoxicillin. This is a general antibiotic. Normally, a patient would take one pill, three times a day, for a week or ten days. I only had ten pills.

I took the amoxicillin twice a day for five days. It was working as it took away some of the secondary infections; such as infected gums. Meanwhile, I continued to try to locate some Gentamicin. Nobody had any.

Towards the end of my regimen with the amoxicillin, I acquired Clyndamicin. Here I was supposed to take one pill, three times a day, for ten days. But I did not have 30 pills; I only had 21. So I opted to try the twice daily route. And that went well until around the sixth day. At that time I started feeling worse.

On the seventh day, I decided to quit taking the Clyndamicin. I had drawn the conclusion that drugs do not work the same on all people. Whereas most people would have continued taking the drug, I knew that it was pointless. Generally speaking, if your drug starts making you sicker, you are probably having a bad reaction to it. In english, it usually signals that you are now allergic to it because whatever you were trying to kill has died and it is attacking healthy cells.

You never hear that part of the story. Doctors always tell you to keep taking the drug...even if you feel better. They are especially adept at this part of the instruction. And I suppose that it is wise not to educate people too much. Why? Most people might be getting sick from something other than the meds. Thinking they are developing an allergy to the medication(s), they might mistakenly stop taking their meds before the meds could effect a cure.

I know, for a fact, that I was having an allergic reaction to the Clyndamicin because it had already killed everything that it was designed to subdue. For one thing, the only reason I was able to obtain the pills in the first place was because the former owner had a reaction to them.

Doctors, are you paying attention? Sometimes your patients are reacting to drugs because they do not have whatever it is that the drug is supposed to be after. It is worth consideration.

Does that always work that way? I do not know. However, I had a bad reaction to Leavequin many years ago. More recently, I had an affliction that required I take a form of the Leavequin. I gave the doctor the nod and we ran with it. For most of the treatment, it went exactly as planned. At the point that it started making me feel worse, I stopped taking it. The drug had done its job and I'm here to tell you about it.

Not everything is written in textbooks. Sometimes you have to inject a little bit of common sense. Either you have it, or you do not. Fischl doesn't.

If I had been forced to rely on Fischl, I would have died long ago. Not only couldn't I get treated for covid, I couldn't get treated for bronchitis...and I had made his job easier by requesting Gentamicin. In an inhaler, no less. And guess what? Yep, the inhaler/nebulizer was created specifically to deal with bronchitis and the upper respiratory infection of which I was struggling.

Let's digress for a minute, by returning to the preceding chapter, and reading about some of the test results. I had high hematocrit, high red blood cell count, and high carbon dioxide. These three reveal that I was having difficulty breathing. In fact, going back and looking at the tests, they even pinpointed the bronchitis of which I would ultimately succumb to. All were ignored by Fischl.

For all of 2020, until around December 24, I would suffer from symptoms collectively called long covid. Most of the symptoms went away after I received a pneumonia vaccine on December 17, 2020. I highly recommend that people forget the covid vaccine and get the pneumonia one. It saved my life.

On December 17, 2020, my new doctor, Fiorella Saavedra, ordered multiple tests. One of those was the CBC. It revealed that my red blood cell count was high, my hematocrit was high, my RDW was high, and my absolute monocytes were high. Those things pointed to a bacterial infection of some sort.

A normal range for red cell distribution width (RDW) is 12.2 to 16.1 percent in adult females and 11.8 to 14.5 percent in adult males. If you score outside this range, you could have a nutrient deficiency, infection, or other disorder. However, even at normal RDW levels, you may still have a medical condition.

By June of 2021, my health had deteriorated so bad that I was losing weight, throwing up, dazed and confused, and finally came the white poop. Now, at the time that your crap turns white, you have a serious problem (nevermind the rapid weight loss).

In late July, tests would reveal that I had an intestinal bacterial infection called h. pylori and abdominal parasites called blastocysts. Fun name but not so much fun in real life.

It was determined that, due to the severity of the symptoms, and the difficulty in eradicating them, that I had had these for years. You're preaching to the choir.

Test after test had showed that I was suffering from dehydration and a bacterial infection. Year after year, Fischl ignored it and often attempted to downplay it by mocking me. At least one of those tests even pinpointed the bronchitis that would eventually damn near kill me.

Placebo effect. He even mocked me about the covid coming and going. Yet, on March 7, 2020, at Salem Hospital, they conducted tests that showed that my neutrophils were high and my lymphocytes were low. FYI, these things occur in people who have covid. Therefore, it would be entirely impossible for Fischl, or anybody else to say that I did not have covid at the time I was trying to get Gentamicin. And isn't it ironic that Gentamicin can also kill h. pylori? Google it.

As I said before, I'm not a doctor. But I can tell you one thing without reservation: if I was a doctor, I'd love to have a patient that can, not only tell me what's wrong with him but, also, how to cure it.

So now the question begs: If Gentamicin can cure bronchitis and h. pylori, can it also kill covid 19? The surprising answer may be forthcoming.

Patient to Doctor

When they "fired" me they cited that there was no patient/doctor relationship. They could not have been more right. There certainly was a patient, and there, questionably, was a doctor, but there was a huge gap in communication. It was caused by a doctor who so wanted to be a hero that he willfully refused to listen to his patient. After all, anything I had to say would foul up his diabolical scheme to make me ill.

I have already stated that it is crucial for patients and doctors to have dialogues. Medicine is a partnership between the afflicted and the physician. If a patient fails to relate his concerns and symptoms, a doctor would be hard-pressed to diagnose that patient. Communication is vital to the process.

It is fortunate for us that we actually have transcriptions of much of the dialogue between Mark Fischl and myself. His Munchausen's is self-evident as he repeatedly fails to listen to me. Moreover, he deliberately refuses to properly address my ailments, choosing, instead, to "stay the course" of his plan to make me ill so he can fix me. Let's look at this breakdown in communications.

April 17, 2018:
I message Fischl. "For the past two days, I have been experiencing a very sharp pain in my lower left side. I generally do not notice it until I try to get out of bed or

standing up. I do not have the chills or a fever and suspect that it is an ulcer. But you may want to see me and/or to order some labs."

When I saw Fischl, approximately two weeks before this message, my blood pressure was 164/98 and my pulse was 89. As I said earlier, high blood pressure and high pulse rate is indicative of dehydration. It could also be indicative of a bacterial infection.

Medically speaking, there is not much that can cause pain in the lower left side. Your appendix is on the right side. The left side, if it is in the abdominal area, could be an ulcer. If the pain originates in the pelvic region, the most likely candidate is a problem in the intestines. At the very least, Fischl should have inquired as to which of these two areas the pain seemed to be. But does he?

Not a peep. In addition, I do not see him again until July 3, 2018. On that day, he saw me for BPH, essential hypertension (primary), snoring, and he witnessed apneic spells. All of these things signify dehydration and/or bacterial infection (especially of the urinary tract or intestines). Yet, he continually disregarded my side pain and symptoms.

Another thing that can cause problems is medications. On this date, Fischl has me on six damned pills. At least three of those are water pills that can cause all kinds of problems...such as dehydration. But the pills can do more than that. They can cause blockages and things of that nature.

Fischl orders a Basic Metabolic panel. This is a broad spectrum that basically checks your levels of electrolytes and things like that. It was a test commensurate with his plan to make me ill but, in no ways, addresses things such as ulcers, bacterial infections, or UTIs.

To test for the things causing my actual symptoms would require something like a CBC. This series of tests would show red blood cell levels, white blood cells, lymphocytes, neutrophils, and other indicators that would tell us what kind of infection I had.

August 18, 2018:
I message him: "The Zoloft is lowering my bp. Today it is 94/61. I think I should quit it.

My blood pressure was sinking to dangerous levels--fast! But I get no word from him. The next day, I tried again.

August 19, 2018:
"Just wondering if you're trying to kill me? Bp in your office was 101/72 and you put me on a stupid drug that damned near killed me. Stopped taking all drugs when bp hit 94/61."

It was true. I had stopped taking all of my meds. My blood pressure had been dropping pretty low when I last saw Fischl. While the Zoloft appeared to be the deal-breaker, I had no definitive answer. Any of the pills could have been making me pass out. Since I had actually accused him of trying to kill me (a feeling I got when he did not respond to what I thought, and think, was a pretty important question), somebody (not Fischl) responded.

August 20, 2018:
LPN Mindy: "Hi John, Your message has been sent to our triage department and they will try to contact you today. If you have any new symptoms please call the office at 503-399-2424."

Sometime later, Fischl responded: "I decreased your medication because your BP was low. You were already on the medication I left you on. Triage nurse should call to check on you."

I don't know if you were following that double-speak. Instead of addressing my problem, he seeks to justify his

141

actions/inactions, thereby escaping responsibility for them. "I decreased your medication because your bp was low."

Why yes, yes you did, Mr. Fischl. You told me to take half a pill for eight days instead of a whole one. But that reduction had occurred before I contacted you. If you are referencing your instruction to stop taking the Amlodipine that, too, was done before I contacted you about the dangerous situation I was in. Fischl is so busy trying to justify his existence that he is incapable of treating me (his patient). His message to me was loud and clear: I do not care what is happening to you, keep taking the meds that are killing you.

That last part was sarcasm, on my part. Fischl actually did care what was happening to me because he went so far out of his way to make it happen. Three water pills causes dehydration. And dehydration causes things like ulcer-type pain, panic attacks/depression, high pulse and/or blood pressure, and weight loss. Can we prove he knows this? Already have, but let's look at my next visit in September.

September 22, 2018:

My blood pressure was 123/72, my pulse was 80, and my weight had dropped to 278. Fischl realizes that this is the result of dehydration and/or bacterial infection, but wants it to appear as a mental health condition. In this fashion, he can always try to claim that I was/am crazy. Don't think so?

In the preceding month, realizing that the sertraline is going to lower my blood pressure, Fischl sacrifices a heart pill (the Amlodapine). Now, in September, he is backed into a corner and sacrifices one of the three water pills (Chlorthalidone). Again, so he can keep me on the "crazy" pill...sertraline.

You've read enough to predict what was going to happen when I saw him next. And you'd be mostly correct. Having discontinued the water pill, my weight went back up to 287 and my pulse dropped to 74. My bp was slightly higher at 136/78. A lot of factors could account for the increased blood pressure...not the least amongst them would be having to deal with Fischl. Pain, for instance, from either my chronic back or kidneys, or ulcers, or bacterial infection, or my ongoing bout with dehydration. Remember, I was still on at least two more water pills.

Realizing that I am never going to take the damned brain pill, he orders it discontinued. In this way, he gets to claim credit for the decision. Irregardless, I would not be seeing him again for more than 6 months.

December 13, 2018:

On this date, I sent Fischl a message about my inability to get medications. "Been off all meds for over a week. Senior services made it so I have no insurance. I hate them. Just thought you should know."

February 12, 2019:

No messages either to or from Fischl until this date. Then I texted a reminder: "bp is consistently around 212/111. My case worker deliberately got me off of my medical provider and I have no idea how, or when, I will ever be able to get meds again. It has been three months. Am already experiencing numbness all up and down my right side. Case workers also keep removing me from housing lists or bumping me down. I am sleeping in my car. Happy new year doc."

Can you imagine that? Three full months without medications that were supposedly to save my life and not one person gave a tinker's damn. The very people who were supposed to be watching over me were the very people trying their damnedest to kill me. So who's crazy---me or them?

At this point, I had twice accused Fischl of trying to kill

me. Here, I just accused my senior services caseworkers of the same damned thing. What you do not know is that my social security caseworker misused her power to completely stop my social security checks. On top of that, the people at the housing complex that I wanted to move into had taken my name off of their list so that they could move women in.

I was offered an apartment at a less desirable place, but the man doing the admitting jacked my rent so high that I couldn't move in (I was getting something like 700 a month and he wanted my rent to be 400 and change. No way). Like the people at the other place, he wanted women.

Depressed? Are you kidding me? Who wouldn't be? I had lost my home when a Jewish fella at the Zoning commission used his clout to force me to sell my home and move. I sold my 34 foot motorhome for a measly 800 dollars (to escape paying a 500 dollar a day penalty) and had to move into my car. I had been living in my car several years when the housing fiasco took place.

To put that into proper perspective, a person making 700 a month would be expected to pay less than two hundred dollars per month at that particular housing complex. On top of that, I simply had no money with which to move in.

How do I know he was moving in women? Because I had checked every month for two years to see where I was on the list. When it got down to I was in the top ten, I started checking every other week. For some unexplained reason, I had been bumped all the way down to 77th. You tell me. Why was the building full of women and no men?

Stress? You bet your ass. You have somebody take your home and kick you out onto the streets. Be homeless for awhile. See how you like it. Then have caseworkers take away your income and stop your heart medications. Move into your car and freeze your ass off in the middle of winter. Stress? Are you frigging kidding me?

February 13, 2019:

Fischl had responded the next day with: "are you on any of your medications? Current Outpatient Prescriptions on File Prior to Visit: these 2 are for your blood pressure.www.goodrx.com pretty cheep

irbesartan (AVAPRO) 300 MG Oral Tab, Take 1 Tab (300 mg total) by mouth daily, Disp: 90 Tab, Rfl: 3 (9-15 dollars a month)

spironolactone (ALDACTONE) 25 MG Oral Tab, Take 1 Tab (25 mg total) by mouth daily, Disp: 90 Tab, Rfl: 3 (3-6 dollars a month)

these two are for urinating.

finasteride (PROSCAR) 5 MG Oral Tab, Take 1 Tab (5 mg total) by mouth daily, Disp: 90 Tab, Rfl: 3

tamsulosin (FLOMAX) 0.4 MG Oral Cap, Take 1 Cap (0.4 mg total) by mouth daily, Disp: 90 Cap, Rfl: 3

triamcinolone (KENALOG) 0.1 % Apply externally Cream, Apply to the skin twice daily small amount to affected area, Disp: 15 g, Rfl: 0"

Homeless, living in my car. Little or no money. Cheep? That's what birds say. Cheap? Not when you do not have the money. Might as well have been a million dollars.

I responded to his message the same day: "No. Not on any medications. Lady at senior services switched me to a different insurer in November. Have not had meds since. I'm in limbo with no insurer. Don't know why they did this to me but it Pissed me off."

Fischl's response: "printed rx for medications, and coupons. For Costco. Cash price 90 days total for both 40 dollars. You can pick up here and take with you. If your insurance will cover somewhere for less then take there."

True to form, Fischl was not listening. What insurance? A little while later, LPN Mindy adds: "Hi John, The prescriptions and coupons that Dr.Fischl printed are available for pick up at the Internal Medicine front desk. Please bring photo ID when picking those up. He would like you to complete a non-fasting lab about 2 weeks after you have started the medications."

No further messages. But I was scheduled to see a social worker by the name of Robyn Edwards.

March 21, 2019:
Edwards, Robyn D., LCSW (Licensed Clinical Social Worker). You Were Diagnosed With Medication management [590466]

I think they meant mismanagement as I had no meds to manage. As I recall, Robyn made a few phone calls, including at least one to senior services. I do not recall any of the specifics, but I must have gotten the insurance straightened out because I obviously was taking drugs when I saw Fischl in April.

April 11, 2019:
I sent the following message to Fischl: "Thank you for explaining apnea to me. Years ago, xrays revealed that I have osteophytes at c3 and c4. At that time, it was estimated that the osteophytes were obstructing my airway by as much as 40%. The only thing that seems to help is tilting my head back. Just so you know.

I had seen Fischl in his office earlier in the day. My bp had been 138/73, my weight was 289 lb, and my pulse was 72. According to his notes, we addressed the following issues:

1. Need for pneumococcal vaccination

2. Essential (primary) hypertension
3. BPH (benign prostatic hyperplasia)
4. Witnessed apneic spells
5. Cough
6. Hypokalemia
7. Urinary frequency

Did you catch it? No discussion about my heart. There I had experienced months of high blood pressure, typically 212/111, and even informed him of my numbness on the right side. He never, not ever, addressed that. No messages were forthcoming. No followup when I finally saw him. Not even a whisper. Doesn't that strike anyone as odd?

April 15, 2019:

When I had seen Fischl on the 11th, I had tried to get a disabled parking permit. Though I could barely walk and he acknowledged that I was in pain (also bore out by my high blood pressure), he refused. I queried: "Last week I asked you to sign for me to get a disabled person permit. You declined citing vague inferences. Please elaborate as I do not understand how anyone can continuously subject someone to such excruciating and debilitating pain so unconscionably."

I think I was being pretty forthright and honest. I did not mince words.

Fischl responded the same day: "I was not vague there are specific indications for disabled parking permit. 1 of them is inability to walk 200 feet without the use of an assistance device. You stated that that was not the case. You do not meet criteria that stated on the form. And the other diagnoses relate to congestive heart failure inflammatory bowel disease and diarrhea and COPD."

I had repeatedly told Fischl that I had been using a shopping cart just to get into the store. I told him about having to hire someone to carry my stuff out to the car after

147

the flea market because I couldn't walk. What the hell was wrong with that man?

As for the other stuff he rattled off, how in the world would we ever know whether or not I had any of that if he never tested? There had been no tests done on my heart. Not ever. Nor was there any tests for COPD...and this was despite my elevated pulse and respiration rates. FYI, we now know that I do, in fact, have COPD (brought on by years of neglect by Fischl).

I immediately fired back at him: "Yes and no as regards the question of whether or not I can walk 200 feet without a cane or walker...which was what you asked me. Truth is every single person using a cane for back pain is a fraud. Most with walkers are the same. As for walking without canes or walkers, all could walk 200 feet without it. We are going to challenge the law as unconstitutionally vague. It implies always while a single episode would qualify. Intent vs letter. As for me, I cannot use a cane or a walker because it increases pressure on the lower back. In supermarkets I use a shopping cart. Your degree prevents you from seeing that as a substitute for both a cane and walker. The advantage is it allows me to let my legs dangle and alleviates the pressure on my back.
In addition, all devices are pain relievers and little more. I doubt any of your patients has more pain than I and yet you ignore my plight. There are times when I crawl from a to b. I have thousands of witnesses spanning the years from 1999. In that year, I broke my back in an auto accident. My lawyer, James Vick, sued on my behalf while salem pain center on state st. Did 3 procedures. Are you going to call the x rays and professionals liars? Do they suffer delusions and bouts of hypochondria? Tell me, how many people do you know who miraculously recovered from trauma to their backs?"

Yes, I was mad as hell. Under Fischl, a little old lady could walk in twirling her cane and he would, not only sign for a parking permit, but probably put her ass on pain pills, too. I was, and am, tired of being whipped like a stray dog. I have a library full of documentation, going all the way back to the date of the accident that injured me. Fischl has noted both my pain and difficulty in walking. And I refuse to carry a goddamned cane around to appease some self-righteous bastard's disability act. The legislation is too broad and my doctor was an ass. Let's move on.

May 4, 2019:

I wanted to get an antibiotic for an ongoing problem that Fischl continually ignored, downplayed, or otherwise disregarded as inconsequential. Let's look. "The osteophytes I have at C3 and C4 have cut through into my throat again. This time my throat doesn't seem to be recovering. Can I get an antibiotic?"

I suppose I had better explain this to you. Osteophytes are calcium deposits that typically cause pain. Bone spurs are such deposits. But these deposits were growing on the fronts of my vertebrae and looked like razor-sharp duck bills on the x-rays. They were always blocking my throat. I had a hard time breathing and they interfered with my sleep because every time I would tilt my head down, it would further reduce my ability to breath.

This was not the minor problem Fischl sought to make it. I was suffering from COPD and that, by itself, reduced my lung capacity by an estimated forty percent (more than that now). So anything that obstructed my throat was not trivial.

On top of all of that, those razors would cut into my throat every time I ate or sang or yelled. My throat would swell; compounding the issue. Every now and again, the razors would literally cut clear through my throat. I would experience a burning sensation as natural salt from the sinuses would ooze down into the wound.

My admonishment that I could suffer from a major infection or, heaven forbid, sepsis, was, and is, a very serious threat to my life. But Fischl completely disregards this as he disregarded anything that did not fit into his Munchausen's. His response came the next day.

May 5, 2019:

"I do not think and antibiotic will help bone spurs and local pressure. If swallowung an issue , med like omeprazole might help or we can discuss in person if that would help."

This statement perfectly illustrates just how disconnected he was. In his mind, he is equating my razor blades to simple bone spurs of the feet. Typically those bone spurs cause bruising of the bones in the feet...whereas my razor blades were cutting my throat. Definitely not the same animal. Local pressure? Let me put this knife to your throat and see how you like that local pressure. Asshole.

I immediately fired back with: "That's not what I'm talking about. They cut clear through into my throat. I'm worried about infection or sepsis. It's burning."

Fischl tired of arguing hands off the reply to an aid named Kayleigh. She responds the next day.

May 6, 2019:

Kayleigh M. Tadlock: "Good morning, Per Dr. Fischl Probably should have an appointment but symptoms sound a lot like reflux and would recommend omeprazole twice a day. At least until he comes in to talk about it. Thank you."

She was, obviously, his parrot and lacked any semblance of intelligence. I was sixty some years old. I'm pretty sure I know/knew what the hell acid reflux is.

Lack of patient/doctor relationship? Boy is that an understatement of Biblical proportions. Where was the doctor? Why was the doctor rewriting my symptoms? Why was he trying to make me ill? More importantly, why the hell did the sonofabitch want me dead? Sepsis kills moron.

No further messages and no office visits until July 16.

July 16, 2019:

On this date, I was seen by Fischl for:

1. Essential (primary) hypertension
2. Generalized anxiety disorder
3. Witnessed apneic spells
4. Hypokalemia
5. Chronic bilateral low back pain without sciatica

My blood pressure was 132/73, weight was 281 lb, and my pulse was 84. My bp and weight had remained relatively unchanged. My pulse, however, was on the rise. These stats, coupled with the things Fischl listed as important, all point to two problems. One, dehydration. Two, bacterial infection in the abdomen. If he paid any attention to the infection in my throat, he would have had another explanation for what he listed. But he steadfastly refused to address anything other than the problems he was causing. Munchausen's.

When I next saw Fischl on October 17, 2019, my blood pressure was 138/88, my weight was 283, and my pulse had dropped to 64. According to Fischl, I was seen for:

1. Essential (primary) hypertension
2. BASIC METABOLIC PANEL; Future
3. Snoring
4. Generalized anxiety disorder
5. Chronic bilateral low back pain without sciatica
6. Chronic renal insufficiency, stage III (moderate) (CMS/HCC)
7. Obesity, Class II, BMI 35-39.9

In his notes, Fischl reports:

151

1. Hypertension blood pressure well controlled labs look normal.
2. BPH symptoms, still with urinary frequency and nocturia.
3. Snoring and probable sleep apnea. Would like him to get evaluated. Hopefully at some time will have a stable living situation. Right now living in a vehicle and he states he simply not able to address or treat. Unchanged from last visit.
4. Significant back pain no radicular symptoms. He feels like it is responding to combination of the drink combined with cranberry juice. In any case he is doing better. X not requiring or using anti-inflammatories.
5. next scheduled follow up: No future appointments.

You already know about the other symptoms and their cause(s). Now, I want to address the issue that he states as: Chronic renal insufficiency, stage III (moderate). One of the tests that he ordered was a gfr test. This test is a measure of how well your kidneys are doing. Essentially, after being on three or four water pills for years, he had succeeded in lowering my gfr to 58. Anything below 59 is considered Chronic renal insufficiency, stage III (moderate).

Fischl was smart enough to know that if he keeps me on so many water pills, not to mention the other three or four pills, that he is going to cause severe and permanent damages to my kidneys. So our hero has now dropped all of my medications to just two. I remind you that this is about the same number of pills I was on before he started attacking me.

By October 17, 2019, I was down to one heart pill and one water pill. I was taking Irbesartan 300mg and spironolactone 25mg. Though no future appointments were called for or scheduled, Fischl (probably after I contacted the lawyer) notes "(around 1/17/2020) for renal insufficiency, hyperlipidemia."

January 29, 2020:

152

Fischl had not ordered, nor even mentioned a future appointment. Nonetheless, I was horribly sick and contacted him on the 29th of January. "1st, I have no scheduled appointment. 2nd, I have been experiencing difficulty breathing. It has been going on for several weeks... If not months."

"I suspect that the same pathogen that is causing my recurring UTI s caused a sinus infection from poor hygiene and touching my nose. From there, this pathogen found its way into my lungs. I have the same, or similar, burning sensation in all 3 places."

"A week ago. I got on here and asked for advice but nobody has responded. Kind of curious as to why. I can come in anytime for a visit or labs or whatever. Thanks doc."

I had messaged Fischl a week or so earlier. Miraculously, that message has since disappeared and, coincidentally (wink, wink), Fischl claimed to have told me to come back 1/17/2020. Bullshit.

In response to my question, somebody called me and told me to come in on January 31, 2020. Which I did. Despite my obvious covid symptoms and my declaration that whatever it was, I never had it before, Fischl simply tests me for influenza. Of course, the tests came back negative. Duh. Once again, Fischl made up his mind that I had the flu and could not be bothered to try to ascertain what I really had.

In hindsight, I'm pretty sure that a CBC lab would have shown that I had high neutrophils and low lymphocytes (proof that I was suffering from covid). But there was another reason that Fischl refused to do a CBC.

When I first met Fischl on February 16, 2017, he had ordered a CBC lab. The results of that lab revealed that I had elevated levels of red blood cells (rbc) and elevated hematocrit. So? This is known as polycythemia. This means you have too many red blood cells. Polycythemia vera is a cancer of the blood in which your bone marrow overproduces red blood cells. With polycythemia, a blood test also shows that you have a high red blood cell count and high hematocrit.

My Hgb (Hemoglobin) was at the high end of normal, being 16.9 verses 18.1. It was a telltale sign that Fischl was well aware of and he knew that if it increased, it was going to show that I had blood cancer. His Munchausen's would not allow him to address anything that was outside of his scope and ability to cure. So, for the next three years, he never orders another one.

March 7, 2020:

My condition worsened to the point where I went to Salem Hospital. There they ran a battery of tests, including the CBC labs. They revealed that my RBC and hematocrit were at the high end of normal. No test was done for HGB. Whether I had covid or not, I had a severe respiratory infection and bronchitis. These could easily have skewed the CBC lab. In any event, I had high neutrophils and low lymphocytes, as well as high WBC (white blood cells).

March 12, 2020:

On March 7, the hospital warned me that I was very sick. I was admonished to see Fischl asap, no later than three days from that date. On March 10, I went to Fischl's office but he refused to see me. I was assured that an appointment would be forthcoming. Two days went by and I heard nothing. So I sent Fischl a message:

"I know you are inclined to think that I'm a bit off but I need a favor. Please hear me out. In early January, my brother Mike Atkins was hospitalized with pneumonia. Less than a week later, I went into respiratory distress and could not breath. I thought it strange because pneumonia is not supposed to be contagious. I have been struggling ever since

154

and went to the hospital myself. I have reason to believe my bro and I encountered the dreaded Covid 19. Stop rolling your eyes. Anyway, I think I know a cure. My body is holding it's own because of some things I'm doing. However, to effect a cure, I need a prescription for Gentamicin. I want to aerate it at 3% solution. How about it Doc. Want to help a lunatic with a silly experiment?"

Consider where I was at. I had a potentially life-threatening disease. I could not breath. I was sleeping in the cold outside. Life was not good. I had tried to see Fischl and he refused to see me. So I did my own research and figured that my best bet was to inhale Gentamicin.

Consider where Fischl was at. His Munchausen's would not allow him to address any disease for which he did not, personally, have a cure. Moreover, his ego would not allow him to listen to a common layman. Heaven forbid that an "outsider" would come up with a cure.

Now consider the law. When a patient has a disease, such as covid, and there is no known cure, a patient has the right to try any experimental drug or procedure to try to save his own life. That was never going to fly with Fischl.

Fischl writes the following response: "Covid-19 is a self-limited virus. Yes you can get pretty sick but if you are over your over it. Gentamicin is an antibiotic and does not have antiviral properties. I am not rolling my eyes that you But I would be careful with things you try to do."

Fischl could not have been more wrong. We now know that people can, and do, get covid-19 over and over. I had it in December of 2019, March of 2020, and again in November of 2021. We also know that people are not dying from any coronavirus; people are dying of secondary infections (usually bacterial pneumonia), and antibiotics do work on those. Additionally, I had been diagnosed with an upper respiratory infection and bronchitis. Antibiotics work wonders on those, too.

As stated previously, isn't it wonderful how Fischl can just look into his crystal ball and tell whether or not I had covid? If we have no idea when I got it, how can anyone say it was over with? I reckon it is best just to let your patient die than to admit that you can't fix it.

March 13, 2020:

I again contacted Fischl in an attempt to get some sort of relief. "When I was a teenager, I got pneumonia and was running a high fever. I had promised some friends I would go out and round up turkeys that night. I needed the money. So we rounded up birds and they were given shots and placed in wire boxes for shipping. The next day my fever was gone and so was the pneumonia. Bacteria or virus I don't know. But those shots, probably Gentamicin, had helped."

"My sister and her hubby went to Europe in September for their anniversary. We all met at her house for Christmas. About a week or so after that, my brother got pneumonia that may be from covid19. A week later, I damned near died because I couldn't breath. I had never experienced that in my life. Burning nose and lungs. Like they were on fire. Dry."

"A cousin of a woman in my other sister's church in Corvallis recently died of cv19. See any common denominator? My traveling sister's daughter and kids currently have flu like symptoms. Is there any test that would show someone was a carrier? I'm concerned because my brother-in-law works in a nursing home."

Fischl, the all-knowing, the all-seeing, prognosticator of prognostication, responds: "covid appears to have originated in China, in November or December as a new pathogen, not the cause of family illness in September. And am not aware of a chronic carrier state for this infection, when ill can carry 20-30 days before clearing but that is about it."

156

"Please look at OHA , CDC or Johns Hopkins web site if curious. There is a SEATTLE TEEN web site that is actually pretty good for updates as well."

Fischl is clearly a memory person. He sorely lacks the ability to engage in cognitive thought. He visits websites (a Seattle teen website! Why?) and reads whatever, and that makes him an expert. Without knowing the particulars of my life, and the lives of those around me, he tells me that I cannot possibly be sick. I'm not sure how any idiot can come to such a conclusion when there is a sick person/persons available that prove his suppositions to be invalid. Nonetheless, let's use his logic to see if it was possible for covid-19 to "linger for 20 to 30 days."

My sister and her husband had gone all around the world in late September of 2019. At one point, they were alone on a train with a family of Asians who did not speak english. They ate food that the Asians had prepared and brought on the train with them.

My sister and her husband return home in October. She is treated for a severe respiratory infection later that month and on into November. People around her were getting sick, too.

My brother and I went to her home in either November (for Thanksgiving) and again for Christmas. The first week of January, 2020, he is in the hospital with pneumonia and I was having trouble breathing. On January 6, both of us lost all sense of taste and smell. You tell me.

Meanwhile, a lady at another sister's church died of covid. Despite all of this evidence, Fischl says that I couldn't possibly have covid in March, 2020, and my sister could not have had covid in October of 2019. And why not? He, himself, stated that it can be around for thirty days. Do the math.

Just because the Chinese did not discover the virus until November or December, does not preclude its' being around long before that. It is ludicrous, at best, to assume that the bug just popped onto the screen overnight. Somewhere, there is a trainload of Asians sharing their dinner with strangers. I was pissed.

In response to Fischl's cavalier attitude towards my health and well-being, I wrote: "So I have been posting online that you are trying to kill me by refusing treatment. I.E. I have had a chronic respiratory problem nonstop through all of January, all of February, and half of March. It is 30 degrees out and I'm coughing my ass off in my cold car. I thought doctors were supposed to help not kill."

It was the third or fourth time that I had accused Fischl of trying to kill me. I believe, on a subconscious level, that I instinctively knew that about the man. My words were neither paranoid, nor delusional. When a doctor refuses to treat you for a life-threatening illness, he is trying to kill you, period.

When Fischl fails to reply, I again message him:

March 27, 2020:
"Been coughing for months. Leaning towards COPD. what do you think about Albuterol?"

I sought to appease him. I needed some sort of relief and anything was better than nothing. Unbeknownst to me, at the time that I sent that last message to Fischl, he had already gone to his superiors and they "fired" me. That made them willing accomplices to the evil that he was perpetrating; up to, and including, my demise. It, by the way, is a battle that I still am dealing with. You see, his quest to make me ill went way beyond his ability to cure me.

March 31,2020:
"John Hildreth Atkins would like a refill of the following medications:
spironolactone (ALDACTONE) 25 MG Oral Tab [Mark R.

158

Fischl, MD]

irbesartan (AVAPRO) 300 MG Oral Tablet [Mark R. Fischl, MD]

Preferred pharmacy: WALMART PHARMACY 5368 - SALEM, OR - 1940 TURNER ROAD SE."

As I recall, I was able to get refills for the next 90 days. After that, Fischl and his cronies refused all requests; both from myself and the pharmacy. Moreover, every time I tried to send a message, I was informed that neither Fischl nor the clinic would accept messages from me. Starting in July, I would go without any medications until getting a new Doctor on December 17, 2020.

It is interesting to note that, after I attempted to get a lawyer to sue them, my messages to them disappeared and the following one was added:

August 12, 2020:

"There's no need to wait on hold. Use MyChart to request prescription refills. MyChart gives you the ability to request refills right from the app or website."

"To get started: Simply tap the Medications icon in the app — or click the Refill medications link on the MyChart home page. Answer a few questions. Hit the Submit button. That's it!"

"Need to refill a prescription right now? Give it a try!"

I would have given it a try except I had already been told not to contact them. And I had a letter stating they would not help me. But after contacting a lawyer, they claim otherwise and invent this message. Unbelievable.

December 17, 2020:

The next tests were conducted on December 17, 2020,

159

when I managed to retain a new physician. On this date, my HGB was flagged high, being 6 percent while normal is 4.8 to 5.6 percent. My RBC was flagged as high, my hematocrit was flagged high, my RDW was flagged high, and my absolute monocytes were flagged high. Oh-oh.

In summary, as a person grows older, he or she is expected to require more medical attention. When I first saw Fischl, I was on two pills. He quickly raised that to at least six pills. Over the course of the next two years, Fischl frequently orders Basic metabolic panel labs so he can keep watch on my electrolytes. He knows, for an absolute fact, that all of the damned water pills are causing me substantial damages. He knows it.

After my health falls to the level he deemed sufficient, he begins cutting back the pills to "make me better." Just the number of pills, and especially the water pills, shows the pattern of Munchausen's prevalent in this physician. While aging people usually require more and more pills until they die, I was rapidly given a maximum of pills, fell ill, and then the pills started going away. Clearly Munchausen's.

Fischl's repeated refusal to address ailments that I actually had, adds to the overwhelming body of evidence that establishes Munchausen's. Ulcer(s), panic attacks, numbness to the fronts of both legs, back pain that is cured by cranberry juice, Depression, falling down, confusion, headaches, night sweats, on and on.

Another sign of Munchausen's is the treatment of a patient for things that he does not have. Fischl put me on Flomax for a prostate problem that I did not have. There was no evidence that there was anything wrong with my prostate. The proof? Look at my medical records. Specifically, look at the tests that were ordered by Fischl. Though he has me on a prostate pill, not once did he ever order a PSA (I remind you that this is a prostate specific test to determine how well your prostate is doing). In three years of treatment, not once does he order a PSA. Why? Because it would show that he was treating me for a condition that simply did not exist.

Fischl thinks he is clever in that he assumes that nobody could ever prove my prostate was normal. Sorry bubba, but you lose that bet. We have the PSA tests prior to Fischl, and we have the PSA tests after Fischl; all were normal and, I might add, quite respectable. There was nothing wrong with my damned prostate.

Here, I have established a modus operandi for one Mark Fischl. Huh? His refusal to order tests that would show that he needed to stop giving me the meds he was giving me. I draw your attention to the lab called CBC. Fischl orders one on the very first day we met. He refused to order another one for the next three years. This is an important clue.

In that first, and only CBC test by Fischl, it showed that my red blood cell count was high. It also showed that my Hematocrit level was high. In addition, it showed that my hemoglobin levels were at the borderline of high. These three things point to a condition called polycythemia. It is a potential blood cancer.

Polycythemia refers to an increase in the number of red blood cells in the body. The extra cells cause the blood to be thicker, and this, in turn, increases the risk of other health issues, such as blood clots. Polycythemia can have different causes, each of which has its own treatment options.

Polycythemia (also known as polycythaemia or polyglobulia) is a disease state in which the hematocrit (the volume percentage of red blood cells in the blood) and/or hemoglobin concentration are elevated in peripheral blood.

It can be due to an increase in the number of red blood cells[1] ("absolute polycythemia") or to a decrease in the

161

volume of plasma ("relative polycythemia").[2] Polycythemia is sometimes called erythrocytosis, but the terms are not synonymous, because polycythemia describes any increase in red blood mass (whether due to an erythrocytosis or not), whereas erythrocytosis is a documented increase of red cell count.

The emergency treatment of polycythemia (e.g., in hyperviscosity or thrombosis) is by phlebotomy (removal of blood from the circulation). Depending on the underlying cause, phlebotomy may also be used on a regular basis to reduce the hematocrit. Myelosuppressive medications such as hydroxyurea are sometimes used for long-term management of polycythemia.

Primary polycythemias are due to factors intrinsic to red cell precursors. Polycythemia vera (PCV), polycythemia rubra vera (PRV), or erythremia, occurs when excess red blood cells are produced as a result of an abnormality of the bone marrow. Often, excess white blood cells and platelets are also produced. PCV is classified as a myeloproliferative disease. Symptoms include headaches and vertigo, and signs on physical examination include an abnormally enlarged spleen and/or liver. In some cases, affected individuals may have associated conditions including high blood pressure or formation of blood clots. Transformation to acute leukemia is rare. Phlebotomy is the mainstay of treatment. A hallmark of polycythemia is an elevated hematocrit, with Hct > 55% seen in 83% of cases. A somatic (non-hereditary) mutation (V617F) in the JAK2 gene, also present in other myeloproliferative disorders, is found in 95% of cases.

Fischl does not test for any of this. But Fischl knows one thing for certain, if the condition is not addressed in a timely manner, it will, inevitably, lead to kidney failure (his goal).

Conditions which may result in a physiologically appropriate polycythemia include: Hypoxic disease-associated

162

– for example in cyanotic heart disease where blood oxygen levels are reduced significantly, may also occur as a result of hypoxic lung disease such as COPD and as a result of chronic obstructive sleep apnea. Genetic – Heritable causes of secondary polycythemia also exist and are associated with abnormalities in hemoglobin oxygen release. This includes patients who have a special form of hemoglobin known as Hb Chesapeake, which has a greater inherent affinity for oxygen than normal adult hemoglobin. This reduces oxygen delivery to the kidneys, causing increased erythropoietin production and a resultant polycythemia. Hemoglobin Kempsey also produces a similar clinical picture. These conditions are relatively uncommon.

Doctors say that patients may not experience in any notable symptom of PV until the late stages. Although vague, these symptoms might help patients get help in the early years of the progression.
1. Severe headache
2. Dizziness, fatigue, and tiredness
3. Unusual bleeding, nosebleeds
4. Pain
5. Itchiness
6. Numbness or tingling in different body parts.

From that first CBC lab on, Fischl knew, or reasonably should have known, that I was probably suffering from polycythemia. This would have been very apparent at the time that I informed him of the numbness on my right side, as well as the revelation that the fronts of both legs were numb. These were clear signs of either a heart condition or blood clots. And he tests for neither!

Fischl is a worm. He was a worm that only stopped his criminal escapades when he finally succeeded in getting my gfr to drop to 58. That allowed him to claim that I had stage

3 renal insufficiency. In layman terms, it meant that my kidneys were shutting down. Had I not been as healthy as I was, I would have died.

On March 7, 2020, when I went to the hospital, they did a CBC lab analysis. My red blood cell count, my hematocrit, and my hemoglobin, levels were all at the high end of the normal range. My white cell count was high and my lymphocyte level was low...a reasonably good indicator that I was battling covid 19 at that time. And that could explain the temporary drop in RBC, etc.

My next CBC was ordered on December 17, 2020, when I finally got a new physician. That test, unaffected by covid, revealed that my RBC was flagged high (6.23), my hematocrit level was flagged as high (54.5%), my hemoglobin level was on the high side of normal (17.2), my A1C hemoglobin was flagged high at 6.1%, and my RDW was flagged high at 16.1%. All signs of the polycythemia that had presented itself four years earlier.

Remember that gfr of 58% that Fischl had succeeded in creating? My test on December 17, 2020, showed it had recovered and was a very healthy 78%.

One thing that you should take away from all of this was that Fischl ignored the early warning signs of the polycythemia and continued his assault on my kidneys. While I may have recovered from the polycythemia on my own, Fischl had seen to it that I couldn't. We have now passed the point of no return. There is no cure. The damages done by Fischl are now irreversible. He belongs in prison where he can do no further harm to his patients. We have an overwhelming abundance of evidence that should put him there.

My fate was sealed when another CBC was ordered on July 29, 2021. On that date, my RBC was 6.07, my hematocrit had jumped to 55%, my hemoglobin has reached 17.7, and my A1C had been flagged as high (5.9%) a few months previous (on April 27, 2021). If you go back up to the stuff that defined polycythemia, a hematocrit of 55% is an unmistakable signal that the polycythemia is present and at dangerous levels.

And you think your doctors are not out to kill you.

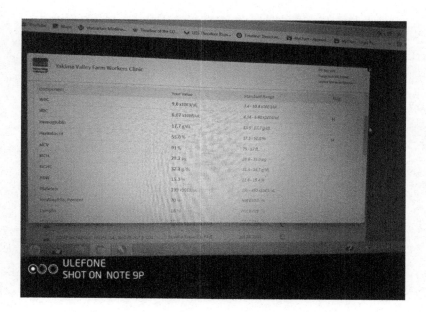

Truth about Coronoviruses

Coronaviruses are a large family of viruses that usually cause mild to moderate upper-respiratory tract illnesses, like the common cold. However, three new coronaviruses have emerged from animal reservoirs over the past two decades to cause serious and widespread illness and death.

There are hundreds of coronaviruses, most of which circulate among such animals as pigs, camels, bats and cats. Sometimes those viruses jump to humans—called a spillover event—and can cause disease. Four of the seven known coronaviruses that sicken people cause only mild to moderate disease. Three can cause more serious, even fatal, disease. SARS coronavirus (SARS-CoV) emerged in November 2002 and caused severe acute respiratory syndrome (SARS). That virus disappeared by 2004. Middle East respiratory syndrome (MERS) is caused by the MERS coronavirus (MERS-CoV). Transmitted from an animal reservoir in camels, MERS was identified in September 2012 and continues to cause sporadic and localized outbreaks. The third novel coronavirus to emerge in this century is called SARS-CoV-2. It causes coronavirus disease 2019 (COVID-19), which emerged from China in December 2019 and was declared a global pandemic by the World Health Organization on March 11, 2020.

* Remember, I had gone to the hospital on March 7, 2020,

and they diagnosed me with acute bronchitis and an upper respiratory infection. To determine what was causing those afflictions required more testing. Virtually everything was pointing to covid 19. Everything.

Building on previous research on SARS and MERS, NIAID scientists and grantees are well positioned to rapidly develop COVID-19 diagnostics, therapeutics and vaccines. These projects include conducting basic research to understand how the virus infects cells and causes disease, and what interventions can prevent and stop the spread of disease.

In fact, within two weeks of the discovery of COVID-19, NIAID researchers had determined how the virus enters cells. And within two months sites had begun Phase 1 trials of a treatment (remdesivir) and a vaccine (mRNA-1273).

Why Are Coronaviruses a Priority for NIAID?

After SARS-CoV emerged from China in November 2002 it spread to 26 countries within a few months, largely by infected passengers who traveled. More than 8,000 people fell ill and 774 died. SARS drew the collective focus of researchers throughout the world. The disease disappeared in 2004, likely due to intensive contact tracing and case isolation measures. In September 2012, a new coronavirus was identified in the Middle East causing an illness similar to SARS. Again, researchers at NIAID and across the globe initiated studies to understand MERS-CoV and how to stop it. Research efforts from those two outbreaks—including development of a DNA vaccine candidate for SARS by NIAID's Vaccine Research Center—have prepared scientists to quickly assess the severity and transmission potential of SARS-CoV-2, and to develop countermeasures.

How Is NIAID Addressing This Critical Topic?

When MERS emerged in 2012 and COVID-19 was identified in 2020, NIAID intramural and extramural scientists mobilized quickly to study the viruses, efforts which continue today. Key areas of investigation include basic research on their origins, how they cause disease, and developing animal study models, new treatments, and vaccines.

The above is an article copied off of the internet. It can be found at the following web address. https://www.niaid.nih.gov/diseases-conditions/coronaviruses

This rather innocuous article seems threatening to lay people in that it mentions a lot of things that are meant to scare you. So let's break it down into something a little less intimidating.

First off, the common cold is listed as one of those coronoviruses. You aren't scared of the cold are you? Well, you may want to change your mind as, according to the government, a lot of people die every year from colds. Actually, that isn't true, either. What people succumb to is additional diseases such as pneumonia and bronchitis, COPD, and cardiac arrest.

Think of that as a bunker-busting bomb. In this bomb, the first explosion is meant to blast a hole in the wall and the second is supposed to go off deeper inside the bunker. In and of itself, coronoviruses really do not do much. However, they can become very deadly when paired up with other viruses and/or bacteria. By far, the deadliest of these is pneumonia.

Purely by the grace of God, I got my first pneumonia shot eight months before I contracted covid 19. Had I neglected to do so, there is no doubt in my mind, no doubt at all, that I would not be here now.

Ever since this phony pandemic began, I have been urging people to get vaccinated for pneumonia. You do not need their top dollar shots when the much cheaper pneumonia shot works every bit as well...and probably better.

Throughout this book, I have repeatedly voiced my opinion that the pandemic is really a scamdemic. I think most people believe that it is a bunch of lies. But too many are scared of dying. We all die. You can die scared to death, suffocating in a damned mask and locked in your homes. Go ahead, if that makes you feel safe. But you aren't safe and it's a waste of time that you could be spending better. After all, what good is life if you are not going to live it?

We all die. Ain't nobody getting out of this world alive. Here's another cold, hard, fact of life for you: more of us need to die so the majority can live. I'll be explaining this soon, but keep in mind that the planet is overpopulated and heading towards an extinction event. And you're worried about a damned germ?

In case you forgot, and I am sure that you have, Wuhan was able to discover the virus because they had patients dying of pneumonia from an unknown source. You probably forgot that the same thing happened with all of the other outbreaks. Remember Legionaires? The 1918 Spanish Flu?

The following article is gleaned from the web address: https://www.ncbi.nlm.nih.gov/books/NBK2479/ It was written by two researchers by the name of Harry Smith and Clive Sweet. It was originally published in 2012. Their affiliations are: 1. Medical School, University of Birmingham, Birmingham, B15 2TT, United Kingdom. 2. School of Biosciences, University of Birmingham, Birmingham, B15 2TT, United Kingdom.

Cooperation between Viral and Bacterial Pathogens in

170

Causing Human Respiratory Disease

Viruses that most commonly attack the human respiratory tract are influenza virus, parainfluenza viruses, respiratory syncytial virus (RSV), adenoviruses, measles virus, rhinoviruses, and coronaviruses. The main bacterial pathogens found in this tract are Streptococcus pneumoniae, Streptococcus pyogenes, Haemophilus influenzae, Staphylococcus aureus, Neisseria meningitidis, Mycobacterium tuberculosis, Bordetella pertussis, and, in immunocompromised patients, Pseudomonas aeruginosa.

This chapter describes how some of these viruses and bacteria can cooperate to cause respiratory diseases which are more severe than those caused by either pathogen alone. Clinical, pathological, and epidemiological observations on natural disease, which suggest that such cooperation occurs, are examined first. This is followed by experiments using either animal models or, occasionally, human infections which prove the case. Finally, possible mechanisms to explain the increased severity of disease arising from dual infections are explained.

Observations on Natural Disease

The best and most studied example of virus-bacterium cooperation in the respiratory tract involves influenza virus. Influenza in humans is predominantly an upper respiratory tract infection; it is not usually fatal, but sometimes the lungs become infected, and this may have lethal consequences.

Most deaths in influenza epidemics arise from secondary bacterial infections, which were a scourge to humankind before the advent of antibiotics and even now are troublesome. The bacteria concerned are predominantly S. pneumoniae, H. influenzae, S. aureus, and N. meningitidis.

171

Indeed, the incidences of influenza, pneumococcal infection, and meningococcal disease show a seasonal association: they all peak in the winter months.

During the 1918 to 1919 influenza pandemic, around 40 million people died. Some deaths appeared to be due to viral pneumonia, since they occurred rapidly after the onset of symptoms, often with acute pulmonary hemorrhage or edema. However, clinical and pathological evidence indicates that the majority of people succumbed to secondary bacterial pneumonia.

Author's note:

I am not going to post the whole article that Clive and Smith wrote all those years ago. I think you are getting the picture. If you wish for a more detailed explanation, by all means go read the rest of it. I may quote some more from that article but it isn't necessary at this juncture.

I already pointed out how the Chinese discovered covid. Pneumonia. The majority of victims of the 1918 pandemic died of pneumonia; not just pneumonia, but bacterial pneumonia. When Fischl fired me, he wrote that antibiotics are no good on viruses; they only work on bacteria. Exactly.

Covid 19 is a marriage between a virus (the common cold) and a bacteria and/or another virus. We know that the bacteria that is the most deadly is the pneumonia bacteria, so why hasn't the media said a damned word about it? The short answer is because they are told not to. There is lots more money to be made at hundreds of dollars a shot than there is at ten or twenty bucks a shot. Wouldn't you love to be a pharmaceutical company making billions of dollars peddling your "cold" vaccine?

The so-called "breakthrough" cases? Here's a well-known fact. By now, virtually everybody has had Covid 19 in some form or other. And the government clowns and their corporate cronies know it. What that means is that there are going to be less and less cases of that ailment. And repeat ailments are often less destructive than the first round. So that is a win-win for the damned pharmacies and their phony-assed drugs.

And, as we get fewer and fewer cases, they get to hawk their "booster" shots. I could run around and inject you with a vial of water and have the same damned effect. But our "heros" like taking credit for stuff that mother nature has done. In this way, they can appear to be God's Chosen people or demigods.

People are so delusional that they really believe that God has a Chosen anything. Stop and think a minute dipshit. If God has a Chosen people, that makes God a racist. Of course, the Chosen people are going to argue that being Jewish is not about race; it's about religion. Liars.

First of all, what kind of religion spends eight days (Hanukkah) celebrating the eight days that the Macabees, or who the hell ever, murdered black people to take a temple away from them? Look it up.

Secondly, before the famous Nuremberg Trials could even begin, the Jews had to explain what made Jewish people Jewish. Do you know what they settled on? In 1946, the most knowledgeable Jews in the world decided that you are only Jewish if your mother was Jewish. In other words, they decided that being Jewish was about race.

If you have a God that is so racist that he would select one color of people over another, you have no God. And, considering that the Bible was written by many authors as a recording of history (and not as a religious book), then you can understand why Hebrews recorded that they, themselves, were God's Chosen people.

Now consider this, if they wrote a history book, called it Holy, and portrayed themselves as somehow special, what the hell are they up to today? Historically, they have been about

173

robbing and killing, they have at least one holiday celebrating murder, and now they tell you there's a pandemic and you might die if you do not buy their snake oil.

In 1947/48 Nasi Jews invaded Palestine (just like their fuhrer) and killed men, women, and children. Now those murderers want you to let them live in peace. Bullshit.

In 1967, those heathen in Israel attacked the United States ship Liberty. They intended to sink it and blame arabs. That way the dirty bastards could get our boys to go to the Middle East and kill more black people. Look it up. Do not take my word for it. All tolled, the Israeli combined air and sea attack killed 34 crew members (naval officers, seamen, two marines, and one civilian NSA employee), wounded 171 crew members, and severely damaged the ship. At the time, the ship was in international waters.

Israel apologized for the attack, saying that the USS Liberty had been attacked in error after being mistaken for an Egyptian ship. Both the Israeli and U.S. governments conducted inquiries and issued reports that concluded the attack was a mistake due to Israeli confusion about the ship's identity. Others, including survivors of the attack, have rejected these conclusions and maintain that the attack was deliberate.

In May 1968, the Israeli government paid US$3.32 million (equivalent to US$24.7 million in 2020) to the U.S. government in compensation for the families of the 34 men killed in the attack. In March 1969, Israel paid a further $3.57 million ($25.2 million in 2020) to the men who had been wounded. In December 1980, it agreed to pay $6 million ($18.8 million in 2020) as the final settlement for material damage to Liberty itself, plus 13 years of interest.

You discount my assertion that the attack was deliberate because the U.S. government and Israel investigated and said it was accidental. Bullshit. The United States has a long history of turning its back and letting Israel do whatever it wanted to do. This is particularly true of 1967. At that time, Zionist LBJ was President. He was not about to let anything happen to his precious Jews in the Middle East. He, himself, ordered the fighters to return to base and not attack Israel. It was also under his orders that the incident was recorded as a simple case of mistaken identity.

In case you really are as dumb as you look, the Liberty was flying the U.S. Flag. Kind of hard not to see that. Moreover, I doubt that the Arabs had any ships that even looked like that one. If they had any ships at all, they were probably dry-docked.

When the ship was being attacked, the ship managed to communicate with another U.S. ship and attack aircraft were dispatched to defend the Liberty. They had almost reached their destination when they were ordered to return to base.

Reminds you of one Adolph Hitler. He made peace pacts and treaties, as well as alliances. The ink was barely dry when he invaded those countries and murdered the inhabitants. I say, if it walks like a Nazi, talks like a Nazi, and acts like a Nazi, it's a damned Nazi.

No, I did not make a mistake when I referred to them as Nasi Jews. Jews are notorious for switching the letters "s" and "z." In hebrew, Nasi means leader. So does Nazi. I can, I have, and will, write a whole book exposing these thugs as a gang. For now, I think you get the point.

Modus operandi. The first Jew gets elected and promotes other Jews to high positions. Then they like to point fingers at anybody for things they, themselves, have done. Case in point, Lee Harvey Oswald.

In my book, A Jew Hides Well, I reveal that John F. Kennedy was assassinated by a Jew named Abraham Zapruder. Dear old Abe was using a camera gun that fired a phosphorous bullet that was designed by the CIA. As you

175

watch the Zapruder film on youtube, you can see the yellowish-orange hue of the phosphorous as it burned through the side of Kennedy's brain.

Meanwhile, another Jew named Jack Ruby (Rubenstein) fired a rifle from the fourth floor of the Dal-Tex building that was across the street from where Oswald worked. That is the only place where the trajectory of the bullets line up according to forensics. Jack had gotten the rifle from a Jewish firm in Chicago by the name of Kleins.

For the record, Lee Harvey Oswald was one hundred percent innocent. Forensics proves not one bullet was fired from the Texas School Book Depository building. On top of that, the overwhelming abundance of records, both medical and testimonial, establish beyond all doubt that Oswald had vertigo so bad that he could not hit a moving target with a damned shotgun. I doubt that he could even look down from the sixth floor window.

But why did Jack Ruby kill Oswald if he knew Oswald was innocent? Fact is, Jack Ruby never killed Lee Harvey Oswald. The whole thing was staged. Lee would live another twenty years.

The question begs: why was Kennedy killed? In 1963, the whole world was boycotting the murderers calling themselves Israel. Kennedy was aghast at what those Nasi bastards did and would not help Israel at all. Not so for his Jewish Vice President.

No sooner was Kennedy pronounced dead than Lyndon Baynes Johnson was sworn in as President. LBJ was a hardcore Zionist and had pledged support for Israel. Johnson immediately elevated Vietnam to a war so that he could go to Congress and ask for money for guns, tanks, planes, ships, and what the hell ever. Had Congress known he was going to smuggle half of that stuff into Israel, they never would have gone for it. But they didn't know. Or did they?

176

For you hard-headed twits who are insisting that LBJ would never do something illegal or immoral, I suggest that you look up Operation Texas. In 1938, Congressman LBJ was busy smuggling Jews in through Mexico.

I also suggest that you read his autobiography. He learned to be good to the Jews at an early age. Indeed, he owed his political success to them. But in his warped brain, he equated help he got here as help from Israel. Not so. Israel only helps Israel. F@#k you LBJ. May you rot in hell.

Am I saying that LBJ got all of those vets killed just so he could smuggle war machinery to Israel? Absolutely. There was no other reason. None. What's more, if LBJ had not done so, Israel would have ceased to exist in the 1960s and there would not have been any gulf war or 9/11.

You believe the Jewish media, in large part because you never get to hear rebuttal. Believe me, there are lots of us trying to circumvent that censorship. You are being lied to every damned day. They want to sell you all the shots they can at hundreds of dollars a pop. I would, too.

So they try to make them mandatory. They try to make you think there may be a shortage (so you'll run down and get the latest one). They keep telling you that there are new variants and they all seem to be coming from Africa. Each variant, they insist, is worse than the preceding one. If they fail to scare you, you would tell them to shove it. And you hate the Africans; particularly those in the Middle East. You should tell them to shove it. Thieves. Liars. Murderers.

But what if there really are variants? Okay, let's play the what if game. Let's say that there really are variants. First of all, Africa and the UK were the first places where vaccines were tried out. Look it up.

The job of any virus is survival. If you make a drug that threatens or impedes its survival, it will mutate. That is what it is supposed to do. Look that up.

This horseshit of blaming unvaxed people for mutations is just that---horseshit! There is no reason for the virus to mutate as far as unvaxed people go. Remember. it only mutates to survive. Stop blaming unvaxed people and sell your stinking snake oil somewhere else. Dirt bags.

To sift through this bullshit, you only need to be aware of two things. First, Jews promote each other. Fauci scratches Walensky's back and vice-versa. Joe Biden scratches their backs. Israel scratches their backs. And they pay Israel billions of dollars every damned year. Crooks.

The second thing you need to remember is that they control the media (including the Bible). The New York Times is a notoriously Jewish enterprise. And Zuckerberg and his cronies are busy censoring anybody willing to stand up to them on Facebook. Beware.

But what about Jesus? What about him? Jesus was a Rabbi. That is Hebrew for he was a teacher. More than that, Jesus was the ultimate rebel. He knew that all men are ruled by either the church or state, and sometimes both. He urged his disciples to preach against both religion and government; especially when those entities are evil.

You think it a coincidence that all of these bad guys are Jewish? Not coincidence; by design.

What about those proclaiming themselves to be Catholics or Protestants? Sorry bubba, but they are all Jewish, too. Yes, they will probably deny being Jewish. After all, they have been fleeing from one country to another for a long time. You would think that sooner or later they would wise up and quit pissing off whatever country they live in. But greed springs eternal. And they believe the myth about being special.

Of course you argue that Catholics and Protestants are not Jewish. To this I say bullshit. All of them worship a Jewish book called the Bible. Written by Jews to promote themselves. They live under Jewish law. And if you ask them, they will tell you that Jews are God's Chosen people. More bullshit. God does not have, nor does he need, a chosen anything. It is just a means to control the masses. Don't think so?

Tell me, when the bastards invaded Palestine shortly after world war two, why didn't we go in and run them out? Saddam was run out within a month of invading Kuwait. Oh wait, Saddam was black and our precious Jews are white. My bad. How could I ever hope for justice to be served?

Jews have a proven history of greed, inbreeding (by refusal to marry outside of their gang), and stabbing people in the back. It would be utter insanity to trust any one of them. And, yes, I know, there are good ones. But the dangers to your well-being dictate that you exercise extreme caution. Do not fall prey to their schemes.

And now we come to the part of the program where you want to know why they are bombarding us with this phony pandemic. You've probably heard a lot of rumors. What's the truth of it?

Ever hear the adage about history repeating itself? That is precisely what is happening. Same methodology and everything.

I draw your attention to a thing called the Great Depression. What was it and how did it come about being? Could it have been prevented? For the answer, let us digress a bit and look at what preceded it.

In the middle 1800s, the Rothschild family had risen to prominence in numerous countries. The Rothschild family is a wealthy Ashkenazi Jewish family originally from Frankfurt that rose to prominence with Mayer Amschel Rothschild (1744–1812). Mayer Amschel Rothschild had once quipped that he who controls the money in a country, controls the country (irregardless of politics). And they live by that creed.

The first member of the family who was known to use the

name "Rothschild" was Izaak Elchanan Rothschild, born in 1577. The name is derived from the German zum rothen Schild (with the old spelling "th"), meaning "at the red shield", in reference to the house where the family lived for many generations (in those days, houses were designated not by numbers, but by signs displaying different symbols or colours). A red shield can still be seen at the centre of the Rothschild coat of arms. It also figures prominently on Nazi uniforms.

The family's ascent to international prominence began in 1744, with the birth of Mayer Amschel Rothschild in Frankfurt am Main, Germany. He was the son of Amschel Moses Rothschild (born circa 1710), a money changer who had traded with the Prince of Hesse. Born in the "Judengasse", the ghetto of Frankfurt, Mayer developed a finance house and spread his empire by installing each of his five sons in the five main European financial centres to conduct business.

The Rothschild coat of arms contains a clenched fist with five arrows symbolizing the five dynasties established by the five sons of Mayer Rothschild, in a reference to Psalm 127: "Like arrows in the hands of a warrior, so are the children of one's youth." The family motto appears below the shield: Concordia, Integritas, Industria (Unity, Integrity, Industry).

By the late 1800s, a book called the Protocols of the Elders of Zion sprung up out of Russia (or so they say). A little Jew named Henry Ford would spend a fortune distributing the book in America. Of course he did so by playing the role of an antisemitic. What better way to get it into the hands of Jews without being obvious?

What were the Protocols? They were a road map of how to take over a country's money, control its businesses, rule over the political party that exists, and take over the whole world. Many people try to claim that it is fake but I have a hard time believing that when a full 80 percent has already reached fruition.

One thing that manifested relatively quickly was the privatizing of the U.S. currency. Abe Lincoln was assassinated because he refused to pay bankers ridiculous interest on loans to fight the Civil War. Instead, dear old Abe placed the responsibility of printing money squarely in the hands of the Treasury (government). It was one of the few times that anybody adhered to the Constitution.

Green backs became the currency of the land in the 1860s as the Treasury department cranked them out. Imagine that, a war was going on and the Jews were not profiting from it. Small wonder they conspired to murder Lincoln.

In 1913, thanks to the Rothschilds and numerous meetings at Jekyl Island (look that up), the Jews came up with the Federal Reserve Act. This Act, entirely unconstitutional, put our money squarely in the hands of Jewish banks calling themselves the Federal Reserve bank(s). Thank you Woodrow frigging Wilson.

To distract attention away from the crimes they were committing, a little thing called World War One sprung up in 1914. People had something more to worry about than who was printing money. Wink-wink.

It was inevitable that the United States would be caught up in the great war, as it was then known. And wars cost money. Therefore, Mr. Wilson and company called upon the Federal Reserve to print up some money so the government could borrow it. Print up?

Yes, they had to print up some money. Why? Because the Federal Reserve bank did not have one red cent in it. It was created out of thin air. And so Uncle Sam borrowed money that did not exist and paid back with money that did. And let's not forget the interest on that money that was printed. Sweet racket for Rothschild and cronies.

181

And now we can come back to the Great Depression. Was it avoidable? Certainly. Look at what was going on. People saw that their friends and associates were making money hand-over-fist in the Stock Market. People tend to think of the market as a business venture whereas, in reality, it is one big-assed casino. The only people that benefit from the casino are the ones owning and controlling it.

So all of these farmers, laborers, mothers, fathers, and all the rest, were borrowing money from the banks to pay for their stocks. In many instances, you could borrow money and buy stocks in the same bank. As far as I know, that practice has since been outlawed.

The insiders knew that the market was going to crash well in advance of it actually doing so. But why would the market crash? Because it was a simple way to buy up businesses, farms, homes, etc., for pennies on the dollar. So the insiders amassed huge cash reserves and waited for the designated day. And Black Friday was born.

The Great Depression was born of greed. The Rothschild creed of control the money had manifested. They scooped up everything in sight...including banks.

People all over the world were suffering because of what the Jewish bankers had done. Had more people realized it, there would have been more Hitlers. And, of course, there came yet another war to distract people.

Following the Protocols of the Elders, we also have the World Bank, the IMF (International Monetary Fund), the United Nations, WHO, CDC, and a little pile of shit called Israel.

In 2008, the Jews were back at it by threatening Congress if Congress did not give them hundreds of Billions of dollars. The threat? To put us into another Great Depression. And so Congress gave them 800 billion dollars. What for?

Incidentally, if you have any doubt that the Jews were

behind the fraud, look at their spokespeople. Alan Greenspan. Jewish. Ben Bernancke. Jewish. Timothy Geithner. Jewish. On and on.

The money appropriated from Congress was supposed to go to shore up failing Financial Institutions. Where it really went was into the various Federal Reserve Banks (all twelve of them). Thanks to a neat law that says that any money deposited in the Federal Reserve (Main) bank garners interest, so it was that the little feds sent the big fed all of the 800 billion to draw interest.

Just like in the Great Depression, they used their ill-gotten gains to buy up all of their competitors. For example, Washington Mutual was a very solvent banking system in the Pacific Northwest. However, another Jewish law states that all banks must have a certain percentage of cash to every dollar of loans (viewed as a deficit). Had the Fed done what Congress mandated, Washington Mutual and all of the rest would have remained in compliance.

How nice that you can bankrupt someone merely by disobeying the law that says you have to pay them. And yet they wonder why the world hates Jews.

And now we come to the ten trillion dollar question: Why did they craft this phony pandemic? What is the end result, or expected outcome of all of this?

You have, no doubt, heard of a Ponzi Scheme. Well, that is what the Federal Reserve system is...one giant Ponzi Scheme. It was created out of thin air. It subsists on borrowed money to pay for all the money they printed. Only problem is, like all Ponzi schemes, they eventually get so big that they must collapse and leave unsuspecting fools holding the bag.

Seriously? What the hell does that have to do with a pandemic? Wake up. They started how many wars as a diversion from what they were doing? The pandemic is yet another diversion. They are hoping that history records that

183

the Ponzi scheme burst because of the damage the pandemic did to our economy and the economies of the world.

I hope that I put that in plain enough language for you. Very soon, maybe even by the time this book gains momentum, the markets will tumble, economies will crumble, and our money will be as worthless as the bastards that printed it.

Go ahead and shake your head. Deny it. Tell yourself that I am a delusional, irrational, insignificant, speck of dust. But whatever else you do, watch. It is coming. And how do I know all of this?

I am God's Chosen One.

* In answer to the question, does Gentamicin actually stop covid 19, let me expound. Clive and Smith showed us that the most deadly afflictions occur when a virus (coronavirus) pairs up with a bacteria; in this case, pneumonia, influenza, listeria, etc. Very few drugs exist to fight viruses. However, there are a great many antibiotics out there that destroy bacterium. Instead of trying to kill the groom, we should be killing the bride. And yes, Gentamicin, the very drug I requested, kills bacteria.

But what about their assertion that two viruses can pair up and do the same...or worse? Okay, let's address that.

A virus is typically RNA. Your DNA tells RNA what to do and it goes out and finds soldiers to do that with. Think of DNA as the General, RNA as the Lieutenant, and bacteria as the Sergeants. Your cells are the foot soldiers. When bacteria are approached by RNA, they assume that the RNA was sent by the general (DNA). It is a false assumption. And it results in an alien assault on your body's defenses. Pretty easy to understand. Right?

But what about the marriage of two viruses? How does that work?

184

Think of those viruses as a menage et trois. Two very different RNA viruses approach a bacteria from opposite sides and burrow in. This arrangement then encounters the foot soldiers and try to burrow into the cells. In such a scenario, the marriage causes the death and/or deformity of both the cell and the bacterium. Think of it as a cluster bomb that can mutate into damned near anything. Variants.

Now, if you have a DNA virus burrowing into a bacterium that is being assaulted by an RNA virus, what happens? In the natural order of things, the General should win the argument either by restructuring the RNA or by causing the bacteria to disregard the Lieutenant.

And now we come to mRNA vaccines. Remember what happens when you have more than one Lieutenant? When you throw another Lieutenant into the mix, the result is always going to be more variants. If three Lieutenants attack the same bacterium at the same time, the cell either dies or it mutates. In any event, it weakens all three Lieutenants...unless there is an overabundance of the wrong kinds of bacteria in your body, then a war breaks out as they each turn to other cells.

And now you know more than all of the researchers in the world, combined. It's called common sense Natural Order/Selection. No, not Darwinism; deeper.

Why You Must Die

I have already exposed doctors for deliberately making people sick while other doctors purposely kill them. Money makes men do all manner of things---usually both despicable and disgusting. It is more common than people like to believe...and so it goes unabated.

Most doctors adhere to criminal acts on a somewhat lesser level. Instead of killing you, they merely say that you died of covid 19 and "underlying conditions." You see, if they said that those underlying conditions were mostly pneumonia, you'd wake up and go get the pneumonia shot instead of their snake oil. Can't make money if they don't sell you something or, where the government is concerned, simply say that your patients died of covid 19.

I have already explained why they created a phony pandemic (so they can collapse the economy and start printing new money). I must give you sufficient warning here. For this lesson, we shall borrow from history. During world war two, the German Deutschmark suffered from severe inflation and collapsed. So?

In one example, a man had sold his farm for a rather substantial profit. Let's say a million Deutschmarks. Almost overnight, the money tanked. A few days after selling his beloved farm, the man was left holding a bag full of worthless money. A million Deutschmark would not buy the man a cup of coffee.

When the Jews crashed the economy in the Great Depression, they were able to buy up distressed properties for pennies. Not only that, they did it with phony money. Let me explain.

At that period in American history, there were two types of currency in circulation. The actual government money, actually printed up by the U.S. Treasury, consisted of "silver certificates" and "gold certificates." The silver certificates were good for silver dollars. Regardless of its year of minting or mint mark, a Morgan Silver Dollar will weigh around 26.73 grams and contain a total silver weight of .7734 Troy Ounces.

The following is taken from Wikipedia. It is an appropriate summation of what was transpiring as regarded paper money.

"The Coinage Act of 1873 or Mint Act of 1873, 17 Stat. 424, was a general revision of the laws relating to the Mint of the United States. In abolishing the right of holders of silver bullion to have their metal struck into fully legal tender dollar coins, it ended bimetallism in the United States, placing the nation firmly on the gold standard. Because of this, the act became contentious in later years, and was denounced by some as the "Crime of '73".

By 1869, the Mint Act of 1837 was deemed outdated, and Treasury Secretary George Boutwell had Deputy Comptroller of the Currency John Jay Knox undertake a draft of a revised law, which was introduced into Congress by Ohio Senator John Sherman. Due to the high price of silver, little of that metal was presented at the Mint, but Knox and others foresaw that development of the Comstock Lode and other rich silver-mining areas would lower the price, causing large quantities of silver dollars to be struck and the gold standard to be endangered. During the almost three years the bill was pending before Congress, it was rarely mentioned that it

188

would end bimetallism, though this was not concealed. Congressmen instead debated other provisions. The legislation, in addition to ending the production of the silver dollar, abolished three low-denomination coins. The bill became the Act of February 12, 1873, with the signature of President Ulysses S. Grant.

When silver prices dropped in 1876, producers sought to have their bullion struck at the Mint, only to learn that this was no longer possible. The matter became a major political controversy that lasted the remainder of the century, pitting those who valued the deflationary gold standard against those who believed free coinage of silver to be necessary for economic prosperity. Accusations were made that the passage of the act had been secured through corruption, though there is little evidence of this. The gold standard was explicitly enacted into law in 1900, and was completely abandoned by the U.S. in 1971."

I am going to interupt for a moment to remind you about the Federal Reserve Act. The Act gave Jews complete control of American currency. When it was signed into law by Woodrow Wilson in 1913, there was no such entity as a Federal Reserve bank.

The Federal Reserve System (also known as the Federal Reserve or simply the Fed) is the central banking system of the United States of America. It was created on December 23, 1913, with the enactment of the Federal Reserve Act, after a series of financial panics (particularly the panic of 1907) led to the desire for central control of the monetary system in order to alleviate financial crises. Over the years, events such as the Great Depression in the 1930s and the Great Recession during the 2000s have led to the expansion of the roles and responsibilities of the Federal Reserve System.

See how easy it was to take over a country's money and,

189

hence, it's entire economy? All they had to do was manipulate money and stock markets. After creating panics, they said, "trust us, we can fix this." Yes, indeed. That's why they forced America, and the world, into the Great Depression.

It should never have placed control of our money in the hands of street thugs. Certainly, at the point where it all collapsed (the depression), it should have been disbanded and control of the money returned to the Treasury/government. Let's see what these thieving Jews did next.

"Gold certificates started at $5 and were (after 1913) Federal Reserve Notes. The obligation printed on the note at that time was for redemption for $5 in gold coin at a Federal Reserve or member bank. The convertibility of currency for gold ended, by Presidential decree, in 1933.

Silver certificates were issued between 1878 and 1964 in the United States as part of its circulation of paper currency. They were produced in response to silver agitation by citizens who were angered by the Fourth Coinage Act, which had effectively placed the United States on a gold standard. The certificates were initially redeemable for their face value of silver dollar coins and later (for one year – 24 June 1967 to 24 June 1968) in raw silver bullion. Since 1968 they have been redeemable only in Federal Reserve Notes and are thus obsolete, but still valid legal tender at their face value."

See how the clever bastards seized ever more power over us? And did you see how they screwed us afterwards? You didn't?

When the fed was created in 1913, there were no federal reserve banks. No banks meant that there was no money in said banks. In order to take control, Jews threw up shingles and built buildings, and then took possession of all the gold and silver coins minted by the treasury.

In order to convince people to accept their phony money, they had to say that it was backed by gold. As more and more customers came in and deposited silver and gold coins, the Fed replaced them with paper currency. This allowed them to print up phony money and hoard gold and silver.

In 1933, another Jewish President, named Franklin Delano Roosevelt, instantly made the Federal Reserve banks wealthy by decreeing that U.S. money was no longer backed by gold. Very few patrons actually cashed in the gold and silver certificates; other than by daily business transactions. And so it was easy to just burn the gold and silver certificates and replace them with phony money (not backed by a damned thing).

What a sweet racket. You start with nothing. Next thing you know, the government gives you all of their gold and silver. All you have to do is promise to pay it back. But then a Jewish cohort signs into law a decree that says you don't have to give the gold and silver back. Nice.

Before getting back on topic, I would like to add to something I said in the very beginning of this book. Looking month to month and year to year, there was no spike in deaths in any country, but particularly the United States, Italy, and China. But what about he world? Any spikes in death for the entire world. Surely if there is a pandemic, there should be a spike somewhere.

https://knoema.com/atlas/World/Death-rate?mode=amp&fbclid=IwAR2Thp3ALwoCV9moAHe3oiLeJ82Wj5oLevmcl6jwnh5ABAQKu-jvF5ftf5M

At the abovesaid website, the worldwide death toll from all deaths was 7.6 per every 1000 people for 2020. It was unchanged from the preceding year. Look it up. If no increase in deaths, there is no pandemic.

So they obviously invented a pandemic during cold and flu season, scared the hell out of everyone, and locked up all the mom and pop stores but left their giant corporate stores open. And those companies posted extraordinary profits while mom and pop filed bankruptcy. I have a very low opinion of Jews as a whole. Even more once I realized how fake they are.

Let's look at the definition of semitism before you get around to calling me antisemitic (which I am and am not). Semitic, according to Webster's: of, relating to, or constituting a subfamily of the Afro-Asiatic language family that includes Hebrew, Aramaic, Arabic, and Amharic. 2 : of, relating to, or characteristic of the Semites. 3 : jewish.

I will bet you that you completely missed what they did. Semitic referred to all afro-asiatic families. Afro refers to blacks (and especially Africa). Asiatic, as we all know, refers to Chinese, Japanese, Korean, etc. But then the Jews weasled their way into the dictionary which, of course, they publish, and claim that it also included Hebrews. Finally, years later, they upped it to include all Jews. Excuse me.

Semitic people were all Asians and Africans. Did that include Hebrews? Only if Hebrews were either Asian or black. So why would Jews want to be included in that list? Because they are trying to make you think that the Biblical Jews were blacks and, as such, indigenous to the region. Only Jews were not black; they were white people who marched into Africa and tried to subdue the blacks. Hence, Jew is synonymous with POW. That is what they were called. And they owned no part of Africa---ever.

I am absolutely not against blacks or Asians. In this sense, I am not antisemitic. However, if you are going to throw Jews into the mix, hell yes I am antisemitic. And you should be, too. No group of people should thunk themselves so special that they are above the laws the rest of us abide by. No more privileges. And stop this bullshit about the goddamned holocaust already.

Stop moving into neighborhoods and then claiming that those neighborhoods belong to you. And for crying out loud stop the propaganda that you are somehow God's Chosen People. A true God has no need for a Chosen anything. You aren't special and, considering the rate at which you pillage, plunder, murder, extort, etc., I'd have to say that if God chose you, it was for target practice by decent and holy people.

Jews have a long and protracted history of moving in and taking over. It is the number one trait that makes country after country run them out. Look at what they did with World War Two. Chances are the only thing you remember about that war is something called the Holocaust. It never happened.

Starting in the 1930s, Germany was starving. To make it worse, Jews posted a full page ad in the New York Times in August of 1933, calling on the world to boycott Germany. Since 80 percent of German goods, including food, was imported, the boycott, asked for by the Jews, starved the entire country.

At this point in German history, the Germans repaid the Jews by boycotting all Jewish shops, stores, and such. But you never get to hear this side of the story.

From there, Jews invented the story of the holocaust. Sure, Jews were rounded up and interred in concentration camps. And many died there. But the same thing can be said of non-Jews and allied soldiers (POWs). All were treated the same. Poor Jews my ass.

The Germans did not have anything to eat. I can tell you, when a man cannot feed his family, he will find a way...no matter what. And don't, for even one minute, ever suppose that the Germans did not know about the ad posted by Jews in America. Of course the Jews feel special and so they should not be punished, or even accept blame, for their actions. Damned Nazis.

Damned Jews. Nazis were starving. It was inevitable that they would invade other countries. They needed food. And so what if they took a few trinkets along the way?

One truism that I have found in my own life is that people rarely do anything for no reason. To sit here day after day, listening to criminals go on tv and curse Germany while the real blame lay in their own backyards, is reprehensible at best.

And you know what really chaffs my hide? Not once have those Jews paid homage to the soldiers, almost all of whom were not Jewish, for coming to their rescue. Jews are too busy hating on Germans and preaching hatred of Germans. They erect one holocaust museum after another as they pat each other on the back for being sneaky bastards. Where are the museums honoring the sailors and soldiers who died to free you when your own people were too afraid to?

If you can stop lying long enough to look, you will see that photographs of American G.I.s in Pow camps looked every bit as haggardly as the Jews. You cannot tell one photo from the other because all were starving.

Look up starvation. It is a horribly painful way to die. The Jewish solution was not simply about killing Jews; it was about killing Jews humanely. Bullets and/or gas would be preferable to starvation.

And did you know that Allied planes flew into Germany for three years after world war two? Why? They were bringing in food. Around the clock, twenty-four hours a day, seven days a week. And many men died doing it. Where is the thanks? Certainly not from the Jews who started the problem.

People are not as stupid as you think they are. Some might take a little longer to educate, but they eventually get it. Am I antisemitic? Not against blacks and asians. But I am anti-Jews. Why? If for no other reason than they are just a gang of racists looking for a free ride.

My apologies for those of you who think they are Jewish and you are struggling to get by...just like the rest of us. I admit my racism; when are you going to admit yours?

How can I be so hateful of Jews? If you could see what I see, know what I know, and listen to God, you'll know. If Biblical Jews were called Jews because they were POWs, and they were, how can any of you profess to being Jewish?

Enough of that crap. Let's move on to topic. Why are they killing you? For the answer, we rely on history.

Whether or not the history in the Bible is accurate is debatable. It was a history book written by Jews for Jews. How it got to be regarded as Holy is unknown to me. And they'll never reveal that.

Anyway, at some point, theoretically, there were two people, Adam and Eve. Even if there were not, we will start with just two people. Now, every generation, the population of the world increases. If Adam and Eve had two children, in this case, Cain and Abel, then the population of the planet doubled. See?

Let's suppose that everybody on the planet had two kids. Do you see the pattern? Every so often, due to childbirths, the population increases exponentially. Got it?

Now consider this, in 1800, the population of the Earth reached one billion people. One billion. Historical demographers estimate that around the year 1800 the world population was only around 1 billion people. This implies that on average the population grew very slowly over this long time from 10,000 BCE to 1700 (by 0.04% annually). I believe that five thousand years would be closer to the truth. Either way, oh-oh. By 1900, just one hundred years later, the population tapped two billion.

Think about the ramifications in what I just said. 5,000 to 10,000 years to get to one billion people, but only one hundred years to double that? That's crazy. It's a runaway train. And it is unsustainable.

By year 2000, just one hundred years after reaching two billion people, the population of the world topped 6.1 billion; or three times the 1900 amount. It's increasing exponentially. Global warming might not scare you (yet), but this rapid increase in growth should scare the hell out of you. Let's see if we can put it into perspective.

Humans, and almost all other creatures, only have a limited amount of space to live in. Our atmosphere, the breathable part (the only place humans can live) is only 5 miles high. Five measly miles. Straight up. That's it. Sorry Jo-Jo, they ain't no mo'.

In case you haven't noticed, people are coughing and sneezing all the time. Even, otherwise healthy, young people are wheezing. It is because there are so many of us that are breathing the same air that the quality of that air is dwindling with every birth.

I know you have heard about the carbon footprint, but do you really grasp its' meaning? Let me put it into perspective for you. If we shut down all cars, all planes, all businesses that are spewing pollution into the air, if we shut down all of that, it might let us all live one year longer. Huh? Like the Titanic, this ship is faltering. It will sink.

Do you know what the carbon footprint is? Each of inhales Oxygen and breaths out carbon dioxide. Remember those words? Carbon dioxide. And not only is there more than 7 billion of us exhaling toxic carbon, but there are even more than 7 billion animals exhaling it, too. Or did you forget them? They count.

Unfortunately, carbon dioxide is just a symptom and not the problem. The real problem is that we are 98.7 degrees. That is more than three times the temperature needed to melt ice. Corporate pollution might put some carbon dioxide into air but very few of them add heat. So which is the bigger problem?

So what is going to happen and what can be done about it? Overpopulation is going to continue unabated. By my estimation, we have less than five years to go before disaster strikes. No, not merely, sea levels rising, floods, earthquakes, volcanoes, and such. Nope. The worst part is going to be the polar reversal and/or the loss of our magnetic field.

Contrary to what Jewish scientists have told you, there is no plasma, or molten, core inside this planet (or any spherical body...excluding the sun. Each of the smaller planets in our solar system were formed when an asteroid crashed into one of the so-called "gas giants." An asteroid is molten iron. It acts just like lead does when dropped into a vat of water (to make shotgun shot for guns). It rolls around forming a ball.

The four gas giants are Jupiter, Saturn, Uranus, and Neptune. Each is covered with a thick layer of methane ice. As the molten metal rolls around on it, it gets bigger (just like when you make a snowman by rolling snowballs into bigger balls).

In physics, there is a basic formula, $f = ma$, which means that force equals mass times acceleration. To increase force, we either increase its speed, or we increase its mass. As our snowball rolls around on Jupiter, it gains force because its mass increases. Contrary to popular belief, it also gains velocity (acceleration).

Think about that snowball. Jupiter is huge, being some three hundred times the size of the Earth. Because Jupiter rotates on its axis very, very, fast, its' day is only about nine hours long. That is really fast. Eventually, when the angular momentum of the snowball is added to the angular momentum of the planet, and the snowball attains sufficient mass, it gets flung off of the surface of Jupiter and appears as a new moon of that planet. Pretty simple and yet our inbred scientists cannot see it.

197

At least you now know how all of those moons that circle the gas giants were made. You also know how the Earth was made. But what purpose does so many moons have? Are they simply there to entertain us?

The solar system is a finely tuned system. Each of the moons and all small bodies in the system, will one day sail into the sun. Think of them as fuel pellets because that is exactly what they are. And if you do not believe that, please explain why everything we send into space is covered in dust. Where does that dust come from...if not the sun?

Okay, I have you up to speed as regards the Earth, now what? Hold your horses, there's more to come. Earth has a magnetic field and scientists claim it is some unknown process at the core. Do you know why it is unknown (to them)? Well, yes, they are idiots, but let's be more specific.

We have a solid iron core in the shape of a sphere. We have 3/4th of the Earth's surface covered with water; not just water, but salt water. Pure water does not conduct electricity; salt water does. As the mineral-rich salt water circulates around the Earth (and the iron core), it generates an electrical current. And, as you know, electric currents generate corresponding magnetic fields. We do not need some mysterious plasma core. Simple science, but not readily understood by simpletons.

The polar ice is fresh water. We know this because salt water does not freeze. Fresh water does not conduct electricity. If you Google it, you will discover that the Earth's magnetic north pole is wandering. Scientists cannot explain it, but I just did. The magnetic pole is wandering because as the fresh water dilutes the salt water of the oceans, there cannot be an electric current and its magnetic field. Go ahead and look. It's all true.

But that is only the beginning; the worst is yet to come. Going back to our equation, $f = ma$, as we dump more and more water into the ocean, we increase its mass, which in turn increases its velocity, which in turn increases its force. Yes, there will be great floods and flooding. But the worse is going to be when the whole planet tips over.

Science says that the Earth's poles reverse every so often. I say that event coincides with the Earth's population; whether dinosaurs or people, or what the hell ever. As more water pours from the north pole into the oceans, the Earth will wobble even more than it already does. Like an out-of-control top, it will tip upside down. Future generations will look back and say that the magnetic poles reversed. Now they'll know why.

God has condemned Israhel. I admonish my Palestinians brothers and sisters to move to higher ground. Forget your pride. Forget your manhood. Move. God, yes even Allah, has said that nothing would happen to you unless you were first forewarned. I have been sent to warn you. Before your children die, Israel will be under fifty feet of water. And what have they stolen? Your pride? Abandon your earthly possessions and save your souls.

For those of you who may be Christians, did not Jesus admonish you to flee? "Verily I say unto you, if they persecute you in one city, flee to the next." For I assure you, you will not run out of cities.

God will not be mocked.

In Summary

It never ceases to amaze me what some people will do for money. No less amazing is the levels to which people will go to feed their egos. Sometimes, like in Fischl's case, the ego supercedes the need for profit. Utterly amazing.

When I first saw Fischl on February 16, 2017, he ordered a CBC lab. That lab showed I had high RBC (red blood cell count), a high hematocrit level, a high carbon dioxide level, and my gfr was at 61. This latter was important because it signified something was amiss with my kidneys.

When you take all of the data, including my high pulse and respiration, it was obvious that I was suffering from, at the very least, dehydration. The very last thing I should have been on was water pills. But Fischl completely disregards all of this and prescribes even more water pills.

As a safety net, Fischl should have been monitoring all of the things that showed up abnormal in the tests he ordered. But he looks into his crystal ball and determines that I will be fine. We know this because he never, not in three years, orders another CBC to check my RBC, my hematocrit, and all the things that CBC labs cover. I gotta tell you, that's one helluva crystal ball.

Little by little, my body began to wane. Before he was done, Fischl had me taking seven damned pills every damned day. Half of those were water pills that were making me sick. When Fischl is satisfied that he has damaged me enough, he gets rid of all of the pills except for two. Then he proclaims that he cured me. Amazing but true.

In three years, Fischl repeatedly notes my pain but fails to prescribe pain pills. In three years, Fischl had been treating me for prostate problems when there was nothing wrong with my prostate. We know he knows this because in three years, not once does he ever order a PSA test to check my prostate. Why? Because if he does, he won't have any excuse for treating me for that.

We have three year's worth of records. Those records clearly show that certain tests were supposed to be ordered but they weren't. In other words, Fischl was treating me for whatever the hell he wanted to and completely disregarding the tests and other stuff, including my ongoing symptoms, so that he could destroy my prostate, my kidneys, my bladder, and my liver. And what about my heart? Oh, nevermind, that's just a spare part! No need to test that, either!

I think you pretty much see Fischl for what he is/was. No need to harp on that any further. So let's see how that fits in with the medical field in general.

Let's start with a simple question. What kind of physician do you have? Does he listen to you? Does he order tests? What kind of tests? What does he say is wrong? What does he prescribe? Why?

Too many people have the wrong idea about medicine. Too many people think that all doctors have crystal balls. They don't. Unfortunately, too many doctors think they have crystal balls. What about yours?

People tend to view their relationship with their doctors as a glorified slave/master thing. You place your very life in the hands of the person calling himself a doctor. But this is the wrong attitude. In reality, it should be more like a marriage.

Your doctor studied Latin, business and, of course, medicine. But there was one course that all doctors should be required to take, but they don't. And they never will. That course is, in many ways, more important than all the rest. I am talking about you. You're the missing course.

Realistically, doctors cannot study you in depth. The really smart ones listen to you and ask questions. It is an integral part of the process of diagnosing you. After all, unless your name is Fischl, you cannot treat a person for what they actually have if you cannot ascertain that.

By the same token, your doctor is not a mind reader and neither are you. Things that you take for granted every single day might be important clues but if you do not bring them up, how can the doctor deal with them or figure them into his diagnoses? Something as innocent as a sore knee or dried skin on your feet or elbows, can have greater significance.

Think how much harder it is to be you. Your doctor doesn't really know what questions to ask you. And you think the little things don't matter. Sometimes they do. Don't be afraid to address those issues...no matter how trivial you think they are.

I had the doctor from hell. He treated me for things I didn't have and ignored all of the things that I did have. And I was too timid to call him on his bullshit. Actually, I was too trusting. I should have gone online and looked at the test results and what they meant. I should have gone online and looked at what he was doing.

Never assume that your doctor is a demigod. Everybody makes mistakes. This is assuming that you have one of the good ones. Chances are, your doctor has invented crap, too. There is not much money in only seeing a patient once or twice a year. There is no money in not prescribing pills. There is no money in not conducting tests. There is no money to be made by not performing surgery. Where does your doctor draw the line?

Throughout this book I have harped about Jews. I have even admitted to being against them (erroneously interpreted as anti-semiticism). True Jews were Biblical prisoners of war. Not one of those prisoners is alive today and it pisses me off that a whole gang exists that passes themselves off as Jews. Did you live thousands of years ago?

I think it cruel to perpetrate a hoax against good god-fearing people. You convinced them that a virus is out to kill them. You convinced them to buy your snake oil, your stupid masks, and your stupid sanitizers. And you got them agreeing to experimental drugs. Holy crap.

In the beginning of this book, I informed you that Jews sterilized me in prison by giving me experimental drugs. So I know, for a fact, that drugs absolutely do sterilize people. It is something nasis created back in world war two. I recently read where the vaccines cause a reduction in sperm count. In other words, the vaccines are already causing sterility. Look this shit up. Do not take my word for anything. Look it the hell up. Unlike my Jewish counterparts, I abhor censorship. Go and look.

The world is overpopulated and on the brink of disaster. If I know that, don't you think they know it, too? What better way to get you to volunteer for sterilization than to scare you into thinking the bogeyman is after you? Look how fast your dumb ass raced to the nearest facility and got a needle stuck in your arm. Fool.

I vacillate on the fence of indecision. On the one hand, I hate the Jewish criminals doing all of this. On the other hand, considering the alternative (world calamity/extinction event), you have to appreciate that someone took control and thinned out the herd. I mean, if you were dumb enough to fall for it, then maybe you need to die so the smart ones can survive. Give that some thought.

In closing, let me just say that I have gone about as far as I can to enlighten you. Some of you will get it; most of you won't. This is a process of natural selection. Either you get it or you don't. Either way, I thank you for your contribution. Good luck to you.

For you bad guys perpetrating the hoax, may God have pity on your souls. You think it got ugly when they stampeded the Capital Building? You ain't seen shit, yet. People are about to get real mad. Your reign as evil white American Jews is going to draw to a close sooner than you think. Blonde-haired and blue-eyed Jews should run. Nazism is dead.

You have been warned.

Made in the USA
Las Vegas, NV
15 April 2022

47553343R00116